O C L
OXFORD CARDIOLOGY LIBRARY

Percutaneous Coronary Intervention in the Patient on Oral Anticoagulation

O C L
OXFORD CARDIOLOGY LIBRARY

Percutaneous Coronary Intervention in the Patient on Oral Anticoagulation

Edited by

Andrea Rubboli, MD, FESC

Consultant Cardiologist,
Division of Cardiology & Unit of Interventional Cardiology,
Ospedale Maggiore,
Bologna, Italy

Eric Eeckhout, MD, PhD, FESC

Consultant Cardiologist & Associate Professor of Cardiology,
Director of Cardiac Catheterization Laboratory,
Centre Hospitalier Universitaire Vaudois,
Lausanne, Switzerland

Gregory Y. H. Lip, MD, FRCP, DFM, FACC, FESC

Consultant Cardiologist & Professor of Cardiovascular Medicine,
Director, Haemostasis Thrombosis & Vascular Biology Unit,
University of Birmingham Centre for Cardiovascular Sciences,
Birmingham, United Kingdom

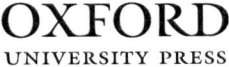

OXFORD
UNIVERSITY PRESS

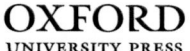

OXFORD
UNIVERSITY PRESS

Great Clarendon Street, Oxford, OX2 6DP,
United Kingdom

Oxford University Press is a department of the University of Oxford.
It furthers the University's objective of excellence in research, scholarship,
and education by publishing worldwide. Oxford is a registered trade mark of
Oxford University Press in the UK and in certain other countries

First Edition published in 2014

Impression: 1

Published in the United States of America by Oxford University Press
198 Madison Avenue, New York, NY 10016, United States of America

British Library Cataloguing in Publication Data
Data available

Library of Congress Control Number: 2013940323

ISBN 978–0–19–966595–2

Printed and bound in Great Britain by
CPI Group (UK) Ltd, Croydon, CR0 4YY

Contents

Foreword

Percutaneous coronary interventions are the most frequently performed revascularization procedures among patients with stable coronary artery disease as well as acute coronary syndromes. The advent of potent antithrombotic therapy has considerably improved the overall efficacy of these procedures. Antithrombotic therapy plays a key role during the pre-treatment phase prior to percutaneous coronary intervention, during the intervention itself, and importantly during the long-term management to prevent recurrent events.

While antithrombotic treatment effectively reduces the risk of ischaemic complications, it is also associated with an increased risk of bleeding. The latter is amplified among patients with an indication for oral anticoagulation due to atrial fibrillation, prosthetic heart valves, or venous thromboembolism which is encountered in 5–8% of patients undergoing percutaneous coronary intervention. While there is robust evidence for the appropriate antiplatelet regimen among patients without indication for oral anticoagulation, data are much scarcer for patients requiring chronic anticoagulation. It is in this context that the pocketbook by Andrea Rubboli, Eric Eeckhout, and Gregory Y. H. Lip provides a state-of-the-art overview of the management of patients requiring long-term oral anticoagulation who undergo percutaneous coronary interventions. In five dedicated chapters, respected experts review the epidemiology, peri-procedural and post-discharge issues, as well as the general management of percutaneous coronary intervention procedures, the indications for and management of oral anticoagulation, and the clinical pharmacology of the various antithrombotic agents. It includes recommendations for all oral anticoagulants including vitamin K antagonists as well as three available newer oral anticoagulants. In addition, the combination of oral anticoagulants, either vitamin K antagonists or newer, non-vitamin K antagonists oral anticoagulants with various antiplatelet drugs, including aspirin, clopidogrel, and the newer $P2Y_{12}$-inhibitors prasugrel and ticagrelor are discussed. The interested reader will find useful recommendations for various risk settings depending on the baseline ischaemic and thromboembolic risk, the bleeding risk, and dose adaptations to be considered among patients with further increased risk of bleeding, such as those with renal failure.

This handbook on *PCI in the Patient on Oral Anticoagulation* is a must-have for any interventional cardiologist but also a useful reference for any clinical cardiologist taking care of patients with coronary artery disease.

Professor Stephan Windecker, MD, PhD, FESC
President-Elect, European Association of Percutaneous Cardiovascular Interventions (EAPCI)
Department of Invasive Cardiology
Bern University Hospital
Bern, Switzerland

October 2013

Dedications

To
my wife Alessandra,
my children Anita and Bernardo
A.R.

To
my mother, she was my life-long inspiration,
my wife and kids Ann, Seline, Pauline, and Tanguy
E.E.

To
my wife Peck Lin,
my children Philomena and Aloysius
G.Y.H.L.

Preface

The subset of patients treated with oral anticoagulation who undergo percutaneous coronary intervention has long been neglected in clinical research. Ongoing oral anticoagulation even represents a common exclusion criterion for enrolment in studies on percutaneous coronary intervention. In contrast, contemporary clinical practice has been showing over the recent years that oral anticoagulation (mostly because of atrial fibrillation) and percutaneous coronary intervention are settings frequently presenting together. It is estimated that 5–8% of patients currently referred for percutaneous coronary intervention are treated with or have an indication for long-term oral anticoagulation.

Since the appearance in the medical literature about ten years ago of the first reports on percutaneous coronary intervention in patients on oral anticoagulation, increasing evidence has been accumulating on this topic. Most of the data however, are of suboptimal quality, owing to the objective difficulties in carrying out prospective, randomized, double-blind studies in patients requiring periodical monitoring, and adjustment in accordance, of oral anticoagulation, as is the case for patients treated with vitamin K antagonists. This is even more true when referring to oral anticoagulation carried out with newer, non-vitamin K antagonists, direct oral anticoagulants for which the evidence in the setting of percutaneous coronary intervention is lacking or very limited. Nonetheless, consensus documents and guidelines addressing the management of patients on oral anticoagulation who undergo percutaneous coronary intervention have been issued by Study Groups and Scientific Societies.

Aiming to provide a practical tool to assist the interventional cardiologist, as well as the clinical cardiologist, the haematologist, the internist, and the primary care physician, in the management of patients treated with oral anticoagulants who undergo percutaneous coronary intervention, we strove to summarize and systematize the current practice recommendations in a pocket handbook. With this intent, great effort was put into preparing at-a-glance tables and decisional algorithms, as well as into putting the management recommendations in the perspective of the general management of percutaneous coronary intervention and oral anticoagulation in the ordinary patient with no indication for both treatments at the same time.

While hoping that the present handbook will be found useful for the everyday clinical management of the cumbersome and progressively increasing subset of patients treated with oral anticoagulation and undergoing percutaneous coronary intervention, we acknowledge we are indebted to our several eminent colleagues, whose expert contribution was invaluable, and to the personnel at the editorial office of Oxford University Press, whose assistance has always been timely and precious. Without both of them, our task could not have been accomplished.

Andrea Rubboli
Eric Eeckhout
Gregory Y. H. Lip

November 2013

Contributors

Editors:

Andrea Rubboli, MD, FESC

Division of Cardiology
Unit of Interventional Cardiology
Ospedale Maggiore
Bologna, Italy

Eric Eeckhout, MD, FESC

Division of Cardiology
Centre Hospitalier Universitaire Vaudois
Lausanne, Switzerland

Gregory Y. H. Lip, MD, FESC, FACC

Centre for Cardiovascular Sciences
University of Birmingham
City Hospital
Birmingham, United Kingdom

Contributors:

Giancarlo Agnelli, MD

Division of Internal and Cardiovascular
Medicine, and Stroke Unit
University of Perugia
Perugia, Italy

K. E. Juhani Airaksinen, MD, FESC

Heart Center
Turku University Hospital
Turku, Finland

Deepak L. Bhatt, MD, MPH, FACC, FAHA, FSCAI, FESC

Division of Cardiology
VA Boston Healthcare System
Brigham and Women's Hospital
Boston, MA, USA

Thomas Cuisset, MD, PhD, FESC

Interventional Cardiology
Centre Hospitalier Universitaire Timone
Marseille, France

David P. Faxon, MD, FACC

Division of Cardiology
Brigham and Women's Hospital
Boston, MA, USA

Jonathan L. Halperin, MD, FACC, FAHA

The Zena and Michael A. Wiener
Cardiovascular Institute
Mount Sinai Medical Center
New York, NY, USA

Gérard Helft, MD, PhD

Institute of Cardiology
Hôpital Pitié-Salpétrière
Paris, France

Kurt Huber, MD, FESC, FACC, FAHA

3rd Department of Internal Medicine
and Emergency Medicine
Wilhelminenhospital
Vienna, Austria

Stefan K. James, MD, PhD

Department of Cardiology and Uppsala
Clinical Research Center
Uppsala University
Uppsala, Sweden

Pasi P. Karjalainen, MD, PhD

Heart Center
Satakunta Central Hospital
Pori, Finland

Lars H. Rasmussen, MD, PhD, FESC

Thrombosis Research Unit
Aalborg University Hospital
Aalborg, Denmark

Axel Schlitt, MD

Paracelsus Heart Clinic
Bad Suderode
Medical Faculty
and Martin Luther-University
Halle-Wittenberg
Halle, Germany

Sam Schulman, MD

Thrombosis Service, McMaster Clinic
HHS - General Hospital
Hamilton, ON, Canada

Freek W. A. Verheugt, MD, FESC, FACC

Heartcenter
Onze Lieve Vrouwe Gasthuis (OLVG)
Amsterdam, Netherlands

Abbreviations

ACS	acute coronary syndromes
ACT	activated clotting time
ADP	adenosine diphosphate
AF	atrial fibrillation
ASA	aspirin
AT	antithrombin
ATE	arterial thromboembolism
aPCC	activated prothrombin complex concentrates
aPTT	activated partial thromboplastin time
ARC	Academic Research Consortium
BARC	Bleeding Academic Research Consortium
BAS	'bio-active' stents
BMS	bare-metal stents
BVS	bioresorbable vascular scaffolds
CABG	coronary bypass surgery
CBC	complete blood count
CHA_2DS_2-VASc	**C**ongestive heart failure, **H**ypertension, **A**ge ≥75 years, **D**iabetes, prior **S**troke/transient ischaemic attack/systemic embolism, associated **V**ascular disease, **A**ge 65–74 years, and female **S**ex **c**ategory
COX	cyclo-oxygenase
CrCl	creatinine clearance
CYP	cytochrome P450
DAPT	dual antiplatelet therapy
DEB	drug-eluting balloons
DES	drug-eluting stents
FEIBA	factor eight inhibitor bypassing activity
GI	gastrointestinal
GP	glycoprotein
GPI	glycoprotein IIb/IIIa inhibitors
HAS-BLED	**H**ypertension, **A**bnormal liver or kidney function, prior **S**troke, **B**leeding history or predisposition, **L**abile INR, **E**lderly, and concomitant **D**rugs
Hgb	haemoglobin
HTPR	high on-treatment platelet reactivity

IABP	intra-aortic balloon pump
IHD	ischaemic heart disease
INR	international normalized ratio
IPA	inhibition of platelet aggregation
IV	intravenous
LMWH	low-molecular-weight heparins
LV	left ventricle
MACE	major adverse cardiac events
mo(s).	month(s)
NOAC	newer, non-vitamin K antagonist, direct oral anticoagulants
non-STE-ACS	non-ST-elevation acute coronary syndrome
NSTE	non-ST-elevation
NYHA	New York Heart Association
OAC	oral anticoagulation
PCC	prothrombin complex concentrates
PCI	percutaneous coronary intervention
PHV	prosthetic heart valve
PLLA	polylevolactic acid
PO	orally
PPI	proton-pump inhibitors
PT	prothrombin time
rFVIIa	recombinant factor VIIa
SC	subcutaneous
STE	ST-elevation
STEMI	STE myocardial infarction
TIA	transient ischaemic attack
TT	triple therapy
TTR	time in therapeutic range
TXA_2	thromboxane A_2
UFH	unfractionated heparin
VCD	vascular closure devices
VHD	valvular heart disease
VKA	vitamin K antagonist
VKORC1	vitamin K epoxide reductase subunit 1
VTE	venous thromboembolism (deep vein thrombosis/pulmonary embolism)
yr	year

Chapter 1

General aspects

Andrea Rubboli, David P. Faxon, Axel Schlitt,
Gregory Y. H. Lip

Key points

- Approximately 5–8% of patients referred for percutaneous coronary intervention have an indication for oral anticoagulation.
- Atrial fibrillation is the indication for oral anticoagulation in nearly 70% of these patients, and coronary artery disease coexists in 20–30% of cases.
- Two to three million people treated with oral anticoagulants in Europe and North America are candidates for percutaneous coronary intervention.
- Both proper management of the percutaneous coronary intervention procedure and post-discharge antithrombotic therapy are warranted to balance the risk of bleeding against that of thromboembolism, stent thrombosis, and adverse cardiac events.

1.1 Epidemiology

Approximately 5–8% of patients referred for percutaneous coronary intervention (PCI) have an indication for oral anticoagulation (OAC). Among the indications for OAC, (non-valvular) atrial fibrillation (AF) is largely the most frequent, followed by prosthetic heart valve (PHV), venous thromboembolism (deep vein thrombosis/pulmonary embolism; VTE), and previous cardiogenic stroke (Table 1.1).

Approximately 80–90% of patients with AF have an indication for OAC, and coronary artery disease coexists in 20–30% of these patients. With the estimated prevalence of AF at 1–2% of the population, one and a half to two million AF patients both in Europe and North America are candidates for PCI. As AF is the indication for OAC in about two-thirds of patients treated with OAC and submitted to PCI, it can be estimated that up to two to three million people receiving OAC in Europe and North America might be undergoing PCI.

1.2 Management issues

Since PCI includes stent implantation in the majority of cases, dual antiplatelet therapy (DAPT) of aspirin and a $P2Y_{12}$-receptor inhibitor (clopidogrel, prasugrel, ticagrelor) is

Table 1.1 Prevalence of indications for OAC in patients undergoing PCI

Indication	(%)
Atrial fibrillation	68
Prosthetic heart valve	11
Venous thromboembolism	6
Previous cardiogenic stroke	4
Other	11

OAC = oral anticoagulation; PCI = percutaneous coronary intervention

generally warranted. When OAC is also indicated, the management of the antithrombotic therapy is challenging, owing to the need to properly balance the risk of bleeding against that of thromboembolism (stroke/systemic embolism, pulmonary embolism), stent thrombosis, and major adverse cardiac events (MACE; death, myocardial infarction, need for repeat revascularization; see Figure 1.1), both in the peri-procedural and medium- to long-term period.

The problem is that, in general, strategies aimed to reduce the risk of bleeding may increase the risk of thromboembolism, and vice versa. Abstention, even temporary, from OAC may expose the patient to thromboembolic complications, whereas that from DAPT increases the risk of stent thrombosis and MACE. Combination antithrombotic therapy, on the other hand, may unacceptably increase the risk of bleeding.

Aiming to best balance the risk of bleeding against that of thromboembolism, stent thrombosis, and MACE in the peri-procedural period, the following issues need to be addressed:

• How should anticoagulation be carried out (OAC interruption with or without heparin bridging vs uninterrupted OAC)?

• Should additional intra-procedural heparin be used, and at what dose (low vs standard)?

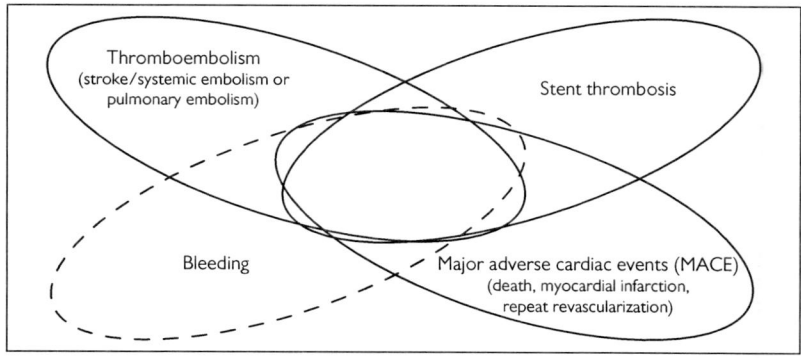

Figure 1.1 Safety and efficacy targets of patients' management.

- Could glycoprotein IIb/IIIa inhibitors (GPI) be used, and with what regimen (bolus plus infusion vs bolus only)?
- What loading dose of clopidogrel should be used (300 vs 600 mg)?
- Could newer and more potent $P2Y_{12}$-receptor inhibitors (prasugrel, ticagrelor) be used?
- Should bivalirudin be used instead of heparin with or without GPI?
- Which vascular access site should be preferred (radial vs femoral)?
- What type of stent should be preferred (bare-metal vs drug-eluting vs other)?

Decisions taken at the time of PCI, such as the type of stent implanted or the $P2Y_{12}$-receptor inhibitor administered, may also influence the balance between the risk of bleeding and the risks of stent thrombosis and MACE in the post-procedural period, when however the following additional issues need to be taken into account:

- What antithrombotic regimen should be prescribed (triple therapy of OAC, aspirin, and $P2Y_{12}$-receptor inhibitor vs OAC, and single antiplatelet therapy of aspirin or $P2Y_{12}$-receptor inhibitor vs DAPT of aspirin and $P2Y_{12}$-receptor inhibitor)?
- How long should this regimen be continued (one vs six vs 12 or more months)?
- When vitamin K antagonists (VKA) are used, what International Normalized Ratio (INR) range should be targeted (lower vs normal)?
- When VKA are used, should INR monitoring be arranged differently (every week vs two weeks vs standard)?
- Could newer, non-VKA, direct oral anticoagulants (NOAC) (thrombin inhibitor dabigatran, factor Xa inhibitors rivaroxaban and apixaban) be used, and at what dose (lower vs standard)?
- Should gastric protection be prescribed routinely, and with what agent (proton-pump inhibitors vs H_2-receptor inhibitors)?

Owing to the complexity of the setting, gold-standard clinical research (randomized, controlled, double-blind, clinical trials) has never been carried out in this patient population. Most of the management recommendations are derived from limited data sets, a consensus of experts' opinions, and extrapolation from other clinical contexts.

Key Reading

Faxon DP. How to manage antiplatelet therapy for stenting in a patient requiring oral anticoagulants. *Curr Treat Options Cardiovasc Med* 2013; **15:** 11–20.

Holmes DR, Kereiakes DJ, Kleiman NS, Moliterno DJ, Patti G, Grines CL. Combining antiplatelet and anticoagulant therapies. *J Am Coll Cardiol* 2009; **54:** 95–109.

Reed GW, Cannon CP. Triple oral antithrombotic therapy in atrial fibrillation and coronary stenting. *Clin Cardiol* 2013; **36:** 585–94.

Rubboli, A, Dewilde W, Huber K, Eeckhout E, Herzfeld I, Valencia J, Windecker S, Airaksinen KE, Lip GY. The management of patients on oral anticoagulation undergoing coronary stent implantation: a survey among interventional cardiologists from 8 European countries. *J Interv Cardiol* 2012; **25:** 163–9.

Chapter 2

Percutaneous coronary intervention

Pasi P. Karjalainen, Kurt Huber, Gérard Helft,
Andrea Rubboli, Eric Eeckhout

Key points

- Percutaneous coronary intervention (with stent implantation) is the most widely used mode of myocardial revascularization.
- To limit and balance the risk of major adverse cardiac events, stent thrombosis, and bleeding, several peri- and post-procedural issues need to be properly addressed.
- Optimal pharmacological management and technique are warranted to avoid peri-procedural bleeding.
- Optimal duration and management of dual antiplatelet therapy are warranted to avoid post-procedural stent thrombosis.
- Proper stent selection is essential to gain the greatest benefit on major adverse cardiac events and stent thrombosis while limiting the incidence of bleeding complications.

Percutaneous coronary intervention (with stent implantation) (PCI) has become the most popular mode of myocardial revascularization. With limited invasivity, PCI is able to improve anginal symptoms in patients with stable ischaemic heart disease (IHD) and reduce the occurrence of major adverse cardiac events (MACE; death, myocardial infarction, need for repeat revascularization) in patients with acute coronary syndromes (ACS). To ensure these results, aggressive antithrombotic treatment is required, thereby increasing the risk of bleeding complications. Meticulous care to several and specific peri- and post-procedural issues, including pharmacological and technical aspects, is warranted to best balance the risk of MACE and stent thrombosis against that of bleeding associated with PCI.

2.1 Peri-procedural issues

2.1.1 Anticoagulant therapy (Table 2.1)

To prevent thrombosis of the intravascular instrumentarium (guiding catheter, intracoronary guidewire, balloon catheter) and minimize thrombus formation at

Table 2.1 Intra-procedural anticoagulant regimens for PCI

Agent	Regimen		
UFH	70–100 U/kg IV bolus without GPI*		
	50–70 U/kg IV bolus with GPI**		
LMWH (enoxaparin)	No prior anticoagulation:	0.5–0.75 mg/kg IV bolus	
	Prior enoxaparin administration:	<8 h, no additional bolus	
		Between 8–12 hrs, 0.3 mg/kg additional IV bolus	
		>12 h, 0.5–0.75 mg/kg additional IV bolus	
Fondaparinux	Not recommended #		
Bivalirudin	0.75 mg/kg IV bolus+1.75 mg/kg/h infusion§		

ACT = activated clotting time; GPI = glycoprotein IIb/IIIa inhibitors; IV = intravenous; LMWH = low-molecular-weight heparin; PCI = percutaneous coronary intervention; SC = subcutaneous; UFH = unfractionated heparin

* When monitored, target ACT 250–300 (Hemotec device) or 300–350 (Hemochron device).

** When monitored, target ACT 200–250 sec.

\# In patients on SC fondaparinux, conventional anticoagulation with weight-adjusted (85 U/kg) IV UFH bolus to be performed.

§ For at least the duration of procedure and up to 4 h after procedure.

the site of balloon-induced plaque rupture, effective anticoagulation is required during PCI.

Unfractionated heparin (UFH) has long been the standard anticoagulant for PCI in either the elective or ACS setting. UFH is given as an intravenous (IV) bolus in a weight-adjusted manner, with or without the assistance of activated clotting time (ACT). Whereas the relationship between ACT and outcome is uncertain, a modest relation with bleeding events may exist. ACT monitoring may be used to show that an antithrombin effect is present, to evaluate the need for additional UFH (particularly during prolonged procedures), and to guide the time for removal of femoral sheaths (commonly performed when ACT < 150–180 seconds). The benefit of UFH in PCI appears linked to an effective dose, although doses as low as 30 U/kg have been used with no complications in routine procedures. Full-dose IV UFH infusion after successful, uncomplicated PCI is no longer used nor recommended.

Low-molecular-weight heparins (LMWH) are easier to manage than UFH, owing to a more predictable dose-effect relationship and because there is no need for routine laboratory monitoring. Because of that and the demonstration of efficacy comparable to that of conventional UFH, with reduced bleeding complications in patients with non-ST-elevation (NSTE)-ACS, subcutaneous (SC) LMWH enoxaparin is currently recommended (when fondaparinux is not available) in this setting. When undergoing PCI, it is reasonable that NSTE-ACS patients are considered to receive a pre-procedural, weight-adjusted IV bolus of enoxaparin. Whether such an additional pre-procedural bolus is required needs to be established based on the time elapsed from the last SC LMWH administration. Also in patients with no prior anticoagulation therapy, either in an elective or emergency (STE myocardial infarction (STEMI)) setting, a pre-procedural IV bolus of enoxaparin may be used to support PCI.

Whereas SC *fondaparinux* is the current standard for anticoagulation in NSTE-ACS, such an agent is not recommended as the sole anticoagulant to support PCI, owing to the reported increase in catheter thrombosis. Therefore, whenever a patient on SC fondaparinux because of NSTE-ACS is referred for PCI, conventional intra-procedural anticoagulation with IV UFH should be carried out. No indication is currently accepted for fondaparinux in supporting PCI for stable IHD or STEMI.

Bivalirudin is being increasingly used for anticoagulation during PCI for ACS. Compared to a regimen of IV UFH plus glycoprotein IIb/IIIa inhibitors (GPI), IV weight-adjusted biva-lirudin monotherapy has been associated with reduced bleeding, although concerns about an early increase in ischaemic events have emerged. As longer-term follow up has shown that small increases in ischaemic events do not translate into long-term consequences and that treatment with P2Y$_{12}$-receptor inhibitors (clopidogrel, prasugrel, ticagrelor) may mitigate any increased early ischaemic risk, bivalirudin monotherapy is currently recommended as first-line anticoagulation for PCI in the context of NSTE-ACS and STEMI. Whereas the lower bleeding risk of bivalirudin is mitigated when used concomitantly with GPI, a strategy of provisional GPI is widely accepted. No indication is currently accepted for bivalirudin as the anticoagulant to support PCI in the elective setting.

2.1.2 Antiplatelet therapy (Table 2.2)

Aspirin is a cornerstone in adjunctive pharmacological therapy of PCI, as it reduces the incidence of peri-procedural ischaemic complications. The balloon-induced trauma to the endothelium and deeper layers of the vessel wall invariably results in platelet activation and, hence, increased risk of thrombosis. Aspirin should be given orally, but may be given intravenously to patients who are unable to swallow. Pretreatment with

Table 2.2 Peri-procedural antiplatelet regimens for PCI	
Agent	**Regimen**
Aspirin	150–325 mg PO ≥ 2 hrs (ideally ≥ 24 hrs) prior, or 80–150 mg IV upon start + 75–100 mg/day maintenance
P2Y$_{12}$-receptor inhibitors	Clopidogrel, 600 mg PO ≥2 hrs (ideally ≥6 hrs) prior + 75 mg/day[#] maintenance
	Prasugrel, 60 mg PO (after coronary angiography[°]) + 10 mg/day PO[**§] maintenance
	Ticagrelor, 180 mg PO (as soon as possible) + 90 mg BID PO[**] maintenance
GPI	Abciximab, 0.25 mg/kg IV bolus + 0.125 mcg/kg/min IV for 12 h[^&]
	Tirofiban, 25 mcg/kg IV bolus 0.15 mcg/kg/min for 18–24 h[^]
	Eptifibatide180 mcg/kg IV double bolus (at 10 min interval) + 2 mcg/kg/min for 18–24 h[^]

GPI = glycoprotein IIb/IIIa inhibitors; IV = intravenous; PCI = percutaneous coronary intervention; PO = orally

[#] In early invasive strategy, 150 mg/day maintenance dose for the first week may be considered if low bleeding risk.

[°] In STEMI patients, administration before coronary angiography accepted.

[**] ACS-only patients.

[§] Contraindicated if previous stroke/transient ischaemic attack and caution if age ≥75 years and/or weight <60 kg, in which case 5 mg/day maintenance dose is advised.

[^] In high-risk lesions/visible thrombus/no-reflow/slow flow/threatened vessel closure.

[&] As an adjunct to primary PCI in ST-elevation, high-risk myocardial infarction.

aspirin should be ensured for all patients, either elective or with ACS, undergoing PCI. Only in patients with established allergy or non-responsiveness to aspirin, should P2Y$_{12}$-receptor inhibitors including clopidogrel, prasugrel or ticagrelor (these latter two in ACS only) be given instead. No data are available regarding alternative cyclo-oxygenase(COX)-1 inhibitors, such as indobufen, which therefore may only be considered (together with a P2Y$_{12}$-receptor inhibitor) for patients who are allergic or non-responsive to aspirin and in whom dual antiplatelet therapy (DAPT) is indicated.

To achieve greater platelet inhibition and more effectively prevent stent thrombosis and PCI-induced ischaemic complications, DAPT of aspirin and a P2Y$_{12}$-receptor inhibitor is indicated. All P2Y$_{12}$-receptor inhibitors are administered orally as a loading dose followed by maintenance doses. *Clopidogrel* has long been the standard P2Y$_{12}$-receptor inhibitor for DAPT. Whenever it can be accomplished, pretreatment with clopidogrel should be ensured to all patients undergoing PCI.

To overcome the suboptimal efficacy of clopidogrel, which is partly due to the complex metabolism of this agent, and the related high (up to 30% of patients) non-responsiveness, more potent and rapid P2Y$_{12}$-receptor inhibitors, like *prasugrel* and *ticagrelor*, have been developed. Whereas no data are available with these newer agents in patients with stable IHD undergoing elective PCI, in patients undergoing PCI for either NSTE-ACS or STEMI, both prasugrel and ticagrelor are more effective than clopidogrel in reducing MACE. Such superior efficacy, however, is associated with an increased incidence of major bleeding unrelated to bypass surgery. Of note, both drugs are impressively superior to clopidogrel in reducing stent thrombosis. Furthermore, both prasugrel, and ticagrelor are associated with a significant reduction in (all-cause and vascular) mortality, which for ticagrelor has been observed in the overall ACS population, whereas for prasugrel, in STEMI patients only. Because of their superior efficacy, prasugrel or ticagrelor are currently recommended as first-choice P2Y$_{12}$-receptor inhibitors to be added to aspirin in patients undergoing PCI for ACS. When prasugrel is considered, careful patient selection is warranted, as in some patient subsets the net clinical benefit of the drug appears negative (previous stroke/transient ischaemic attack) or neutral (age $\geq$ 75 years and/or weight < 60 kg). Of note, prasugrel administration should only be performed when patients are clopidogrel-naive, and when the coronary anatomy is known, although in patients undergoing primary PCI for STEMI, administration as early as possible is accepted.

Further antiplatelet effect can be obtained with *GPI*, including abciximab, eptifibatide, and tirofiban, as platelet aggregation and adhesion to disrupted endothelium is largely mediated by the surface glycoprotein IIb/IIIa receptor. Whereas data from the pre-DAPT era showed a reduction of ischaemic events with GPI, at the price however of some increase in bleeding, more contemporary trials of patients receiving P2Y$_{12}$-receptor inhibitors yielded mixed results. At present, therefore, routine use of GPI is no longer recommended. On the other hand, intra-procedural administration is warranted in the presence of high-risk lesions, threatening vessel closure, visible thrombus, or no-reflow, regardless of the clinical indication (stable IHD or ACS) for PCI. Also, GPI should be considered in elective patients treated with UFH and not pretreated with clopidogrel (or any other P2Y$_{12}$-receptor inhibitor). In primary PCI for STEMI, routine use of GPI in conjunction with UFH may only be considered when the bleeding risk is low, regardless of whether patients were pretreated with clopidogrel. Upstream use, that is, before arrival to the catheterization laboratory, of GPI is not routinely recommended in either NSTE-ACS or STEMI patients, owing to the reported increase in bleeding complications, with no substantial benefit on ischaemic events. Such a strategy may only be considered for high-risk patients with STEMI (haemodynamic impairment, anterior myocardial infarction) who are being transfered for primary PCI, especially if early (2–3 h) after symptom onset. Whereas the combination of GPI with bivalirudin should be restricted to bail-out situations, concomitant IV infusion of UFH and GPI is warranted in all cases. The IV route is the standard for GPI administration, because the strategy of intracoronary administration via bolus only has shown no benefit (but also no harm) for either efficacy or safety.

Technique. Whereas the femoral artery access has long been the standard for coronary angiography and PCI, the *radial artery access* is now being increasingly used. A learning curve exists for the radial approach that will affect procedure time and radiation dose, with a trend toward lower procedural success rate compared to femoral approach. However, the radial approach markedly diminishes the rate of access-related bleeding and vascular complications, especially in PCI performed in ACS when aggressive antithrombotic regimens are used. It has been recognized that limiting peri-procedural bleeding is of great importance because of the negative impact it has on prognosis and the increase it causes in both length of hospitalization and costs. Because the favourable results of the radial approach are also seen in patients undergoing primary PCI for STEMI, for whom short- and long-term mortality may even be reduced, such vascular access should be routinely considered in both the elective and ACS setting, provided that adequate expertise is available.

When using the femoral approach, *vascular closure devices (VCD)*, either collagen- or suture-mediated, have been shown to decrease the time to haemostasis compared to manual compression. In patients at greatest pre-procedural risk of bleeding, and/or submitted to aggressive antithrombotic therapy, VCD has been shown to significantly reduce also the incidence of access-site bleeding complications. Thus, although being generally used for the purpose of achieving earlier ambulation and, hence, earlier hospital discharge, VCD may also be considered to reduce complications at the femoral access site in patients at increased risk of bleeding.

Among adjunctive therapeutic devices, *aspiration thrombectomy* may have a role in patients undergoing primary PCI for STEMI. Given the reported efficacy on myocardial perfusion and the subsequent incidence of MACE, including mortality, manual thrombus aspiration (but not mechanical) should be routinely considered in this setting, in conjuction with conventional antithrombotic treatment.

2.1.3 Stents (Table 2.3)

Contemporary PCI is associated in the majority (approximately 85%) of cases with stent implantation, owing to the established superiority over stand-alone balloon angioplasty on the occurrence of restenosis. Also, by scaffolding the coronary wall, stents are highly effective in preventing elastic recoil (the immediate reduction in lumen following balloon deflation) and abrupt vessel closure.

Stents can be generally classified as bare-metal (BMS), drug-eluting (DES), and 'bio-active' (BAS). Also, the more recently developed bioresorbable vascular scaffolds (BVS) are to be mentioned.

BMS are composed of either stainless steel or cobalt- or platinum-chrome alloys, whereas *DES* vary according to material and design, drug content, and the polymer used for drug elution. In DES, an anti-proliferative drug (sirolimus, paclitaxel, everolimus, zotarolimus, biolimus-A9™, amphilimus™) is adsorbed to a synthetic polymer covering the stent struts and is released over time at the site of implantation, blunting neo-intimal proliferation and hence preventing restenosis. Whereas, in fact, both BMS

Device		Characteristics
BMS		stainless steel or non stainless-steel, cobalt- or platinum-chrome alloy
DES	Early generation:	sirolimus-, paclitaxel-eluting
	New generation:	zotarolimus-, everolimus-eluting (durable polymer)
		biolimus A9™-eluting (bioabsorbable polymer)
		amphilimus™-eluting (polymer-free)
BAS		diamond-like carbon- or titanium nitric oxide-coated
		endothelial progenitor cells-capturing
BVS		non-drug-eluting
		everolimus-, myolimus-, sirolimus-eluting

Table 2.3 General classification of coronary stents/scaffolds

BAS = 'bio-active' stents; BMS = bare-metal stents; BVS = bioresorbable vascular scaffolds; DES = drug-eluting stents

and DES exert a comparable effect on elastic recoil and negative remodelling (the active and progressive decrease in the size of the vessel area following balloon dilatation), only DES exert an additional effect on the remaining mechanism at the basis of restenosis, namely, neo-intimal hyperplasia (thickening of the intima as the response to injury).

Superiority of DES over BMS regarding the incidence of restenosis, and hence repeat revascularization, has long been demonstrated, with no increase in death and/or myocardial infarction. Therefore, DES are currently recommended as first-choice option, especially when the risk of restenosis is higher (diabetes, long lesions, small vessels, chronic total occlusion, bifurcation, and restenotic lesions). Compared to BMS, DES may be associated with a higher risk of stent thrombosis, mainly because of delayed endothelization and chronic inflammation related to presence of the polymer and release of anti-proliferative drugs. Prolonged DAPT (up to 12 months) is therefore recommended. Shorter durations (≤3–6 months) of DAPT may be considered with new-generation (everolimus-, zotarolimus-eluting, or polymer-reabsorbable or polymer-free) DES because of the observation of a reduced incidence of stent thrombosis. Since early discontinuation of DAPT is recognized as the most potent predictor of DES thrombosis, discussion with the patient regarding the need for and duration of DAPT as well as the ability to comply with and tolerate DAPT is mandatory before DES implantation.

In the attempt to increase the biocompatibility of BMS, thereby reducing the risk of stent thrombosis as well as of restenosis without use of polymer-eluted drugs, various coatings have been used. Among these so-called BAS, diamond-like carbon- and titanium nitric oxide-coated stents have shown promising results (in this latter case even when compared with a DES), an option making DAPT duration shorter than the one month commonly recommended for BMS. No such promising results have been obtained with BAS which capture endothelial progenitor cells and are capable of promoting rapid re-endothelization at the site of implantation, which therefore have currently no specific indication.

BVS have been developed with the aim to provide adequate mechanical scaffolding for the initial months following implantation, but deliver subsequent reabsorption of the scaffold, thereby facilitating complete vessel healing and restoration of normal vascular function (which, in contrast, is permanently impaired after implantation of metallic stents). Also, BVS have the potential to reduce the risk of late stent thrombosis, neo-atherosclerosis, and the local inflammation caused by the presence of a foreign body. Different materials are used in BVS, of which polylevolactic acid (PLLA) is the most used and extensively investigated. An anti-proliferative drug may or may be not eluted by BVS. Initial results with an everolimus-eluting BVS, for which degradation has been shown to start six months after implantation and complete within two years, show no significant late luminal loss, return of vasoreactivity, and low rate of MACE at follow up. DAPT is required for some months after implantation, and likely at least until BVS degradation begins (six months).

In Figure 2.1, a comprehensive strategy aiming to balance the risk of MACE against that of bleeding associated with PCI is outlined.

2.1.4 Adverse events (Table 2.4)

Because of its invasive nature, PCI is associated with peri-procedural ischaemic complications (death, myocardial infarction, need for emergency bypass surgery, stroke), vascular complications, and bleeding.

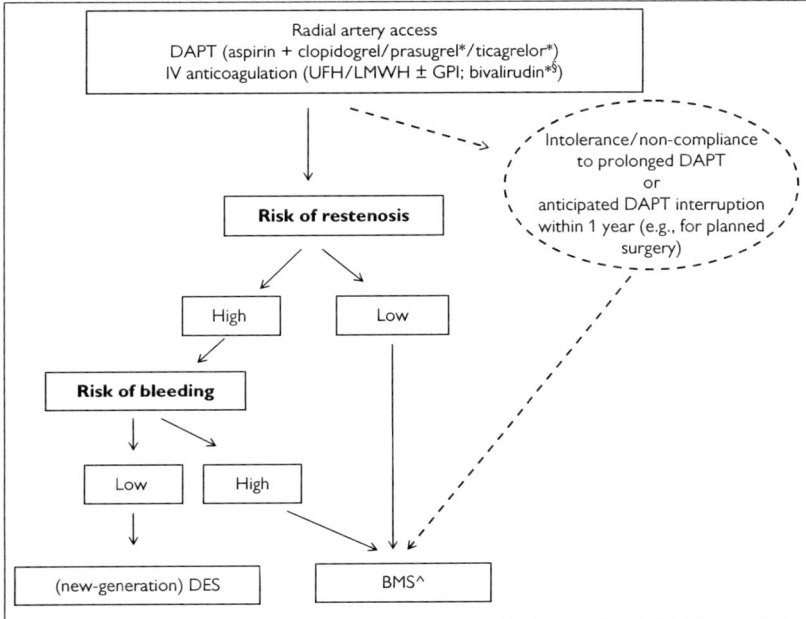

Figure 2.1 General algorithm to optimize the balance between risk of MACE, stent thrombosis, and bleeding associated with PCI.

BMS= bare-metal stents; DAPT= dual antiplatelet therapy; DES= drug-eluting stents; GPI= glycoprotein IIb/IIIa inhibitors

* Only for PCI in ACS. ^ BAS, polymer-reabsorbable or polymer-free DES, or BVS may also be considered. § Bail-out use of GPI accepted.

Table 2.4 Peri-procedural incidence of adverse events

Adverse event	(%)
Ischaemic:	
Death	0.7–4.8^
Myocardial infarction*	1.0–5.0
Emergency bypass surgery	<1.0
Stroke	0.1–0.4
Vascular complications (by femoral approach)	2.0–6.0
Clinically significant bleeding§	1.0–7.0

^ In elective PCI and primary PCI for STEMI, respectively.

* To be defined according to the 3rd Universal Definition (type 4a) as cardiac troponin increase >5 × 99th percentile (with normal baseline values) or >20% (with elevated and stable or falling baseline values) plus one of the following: (a) symptoms of myocardial ischaemia; (b) new ischaemic electrocardiographic or new left bundle branch block; (c) loss of patency of major coronary artery or side branch, slow flow/no-reflow, or embolization at angiography; or (d) imaging demonstration of new loss of viable myocardium or new regional wall motion abnormality.

§ Prompting evaluation and/or treatment, or fatal.

The risk of procedural-related *death* is increased in the presence of advanced age, co-morbidities (diabetes, chronic kidney disease, congestive heart failure), multivessel coronary artery disease, high-risk lesion, urgent or emergency setting, and shock. Peri-procedural *myocardial infarction* may be related to acute vessel closure, embolization and no-reflow, side branch occlusion, and acute (≤24 h) stent thrombosis. These potential complications should be properly anticipated by adopting adequate strategies, including prophylactic wiring of relevant side branches and the use of timely and optimal antithrombotic regimens, and properly treated when they occur. Particularly challenging is the management of the no-reflow phenomenon, which is commonly due to vasospasm, and downstream embolization of debris dislodged by the procedure, especially in the context of primary PCI for STEMI, as a clear benefit on infarct size and mortality has not been clearly shown with various pharmacological agents. However, intracoronary vasodilators (adenosine 30–60 mcg, verapamil 0.5–1 mg) should be administered when no-reflow occurs. *Emergency bypass surgery* has dramatically decreased over the years with advances in PCI technology, especially stents. Predictors of emergency bypass surgery, which is invariably associated with high in-hospital mortality (7–14%), include cardiogenic shock, multivessel disease, emergency PCI, and high-risk lesion. Whereas *stroke* is a rare complication of PCI, in-hospital mortality rate is high (25–30%). Factors associated with higher risk of peri-procedural stroke, which in most cases is ischaemic, include known cerebrovascular disease, use of the intra-aortic balloon pump (IABP), advanced age, female gender, and previous thrombolytic therapy.

Vascular complications are mostly observed when the femoral access is used, and include access-site or retroperitoneal haematoma, pseudoaneurysm, arteriovenous fistula, and arterial dissection or occlusion. Vascular complications are more frequent with advanced age, low body surface area, emergency procedures, peripheral artery disease, use of GPI, and female gender. Although radial access markedly decreases vascular complications, compartment syndrome (increased pressure within the forearm compartment with associated impaired blood supply to muscles and nerves), pseudoaneurysm, and sterile abscess may be rarely observed. In about 5% of cases, loss of radial pulse, thereby precluding subsequent procedures, occurs.

Bleeding is an important complication of PCI, as it is now recognized as a major risk factor for subsequent mortality. Bleeding may lead to death directly (intracranial, causing shock) or through ischaemic complications that occurr when antiplatelets are withdrawn in response to bleeding. The true incidence of peri-procedural bleeding is difficult to estimate, because of the highly variable definitions given in clinical studies. In the attempt to homogenize bleeding definitions, and therefore to make comparisons among different clinical settings possible, a standardized definition should be adopted (Table 2.5).

The overall incidence of clinically significant (prompting evaluation and/or treatment, or fatal) peri-procedural bleeding can be estimated to be 1–7%, depending on patient characteristics, intensity of peri-procedural antiplatelet and anticoagulant therapy, vascular access site, and sheath size. In general, bleeding complications, especially at the vascular access site, are related to the intensity of antithrombotic therapy, and therefore are more common in PCI for ACS, where aggressive antiplatelet and anticoagulant regimens are used.

Bleeding risk assessment is recommended before PCI and should preferably be carried out according to validated scores (which have been developed for both ACS and elective patients). Alternatively, it should be recalled that female gender, advanced age, impaired renal function, baseline anaemia, ACS setting, aggressive antithrombotic therapy, and IABP increase (in an additive way) the risk of peri-procedural bleeding.

Table 2.5 Bleeding Academic Research Consortium (BARC) classification of bleeding

Class	Characteristics
Type 0	No bleeding
Type 1	Not actionable, and not causing unscheduled procedures/treatment; may induce therapy self-discontinuation
Type 2	Any overt, actionable bleeding not fitting criteria for type 3, 4, or 5 but meeting ≥1 of the following criteria: (a) requiring non-surgical medical intervention (b) leading to hospitalization/increased level of care (c) prompting evaluation
Type 3a	Overt bleeding + Hgb drop 3–4.9 g/dl Any blood transfusion with overt bleeding
Type 3b	Overt bleeding + Hgb drop ≥5 g/dl Cardiac tamponade Requiring surgical intervention (excluding dental/nasal/skin/haemorrhoid) Requiring intravenous vasoactive agents
Type 3c	Intracranial haemorrhage (subcategories confirmed at autopsy/imaging/lumbar puncture) Intraocular compromising vision
Type 4	CABG-related bleeding: Perioperative intracranial ≤48 h Requiring reoperation after sternotomy closure Blood transfusion ≥5 units over 48 h period Chest tube output ≥2 litres over 24 h period
Type 5	Fatal (overt or confirmed at autopsy/imaging)

CABG = coronary bypass surgery; Hgb = haemoglobin

Table 2.6 Measures to minimize the risk of peri-procedural bleeding

Anticoagulant regimens associated with lower risk
Weight-based dosing of anticoagulants
ACT to guide UFH dosing
Avoidance of excess anticoagulation
Dose-adjustment in patients with impaired renal function
Radial artery access
Avoidance of femoral vein cannulation

ACT = activated clotting time; GPI = glycoprotein IIb/IIIa inhibitors; UFH = unfractionated heparin

Whereas the overall approach to PCI should be individualized to balance the peri-procedural risk of MACE against that of bleeding, in general measures should be adopted to minimize the risk of peri-procedural bleeding (Table 2.6).

In the event that clinically significant bleeding occurs, IV anticoagulants (UFH, bivalirudin) and/or GPI should be immediately stopped when ongoing, and reversal (protamine sulphate) considered. In contrast, the benefit of interrupting oral antiplatelet therapy should be carefully weighed against the risk of stent thrombosis. As withholding oral antiplatelet early after PCI increases the risk of stent thrombosis, treatment interruption should always be considered a temporary measure. In general, clinically significant bleeding requires interruption of oral antiplatelet therapy, unless haemorrhage can be adequately controlled by specific haemostatic measures. It should be striven however, not to interrupt both aspirin and $P2Y_{12}$-receptor inhibitor at the same time. Whenever blood transfusion is deemed necessary, a restrictive strategy should be adopted and reserved to patients with haematocrit <25% and/or haemogolobin <8 g/dl, owing to the established deleterious effects of blood transfusions on outcome.

2.2 Post-procedural issues

2.2.1 Antiplatelet therapy (Tables 2.2, 2.7)

Following PCI, low-dose aspirin should be continued indefinitely. DAPT with aspirin and a $P2Y_{12}$-receptor inhibitor (clopidogrel, prasugrel, ticagrelor) should be given for some time after PCI to prevent stent thrombosis.

Owing to the observation of a low incidence of stent thrombosis (and MACE) and/or earlier and complete re-endothelization, durations of DAPT shorter than generally

Table 2.7 Recommended durations of DAPT after PCI

Setting	Months
BMS in stable IHD	1
DES in stable IHD	6–12
BMS/DES in ACS	12

ACS = acute coronary syndrome; BMS = bare-metal stent; DAPT = dual antiplatelet therapy; DES = drug-eluting stent; IHD = ischaemic heart disease recommended may be considered, essentially in patients at high bleeding risk and/or in case of need (bleeding, unplanned surgery), with new-generation zotarolimus- (one month) and everolimus- (three months) DES and polymer-free, amphilimus™- (three months) DES, as well as with diamond-like carbon-coated BAS (two weeks). Also, limitation of DAPT to six months may be considered with new-generation, polymer-reabsorbable, biolimus A9™-DES and everolimus-eluting BVS. One-month duration of DAPT should be considered following stand-alone angioplasty with paclitaxel-coated drug-eluting balloons (DEB).

The duration of DAPT with aspirin and prasugrel or ticagrelor in ACS patients undergoing PCI should be the same as for DAPT with aspirin and clopidogrel (Table 2.2). In accordance with current recommendations, it should not be overlooked that earlier discontinuation of DAPT may be considered whenever the risk of morbidity from bleeding is deemed to outweigh the anticipated benefit of the recommended duration. On the other hand, no sound evidence is currently supporting prolongation of DAPT beyond 12 months, although such strategy may be considered based on individual decision making in specific patient subsets (left main or last remaining vessel stenting, long stented segment with multiple stents) receiving DES.

2.2.2 Stent thrombosis

The occurrence of thrombosis at the stent site may be observed at various time points following PCI (Table 2.8) and with various incidence (Table 2.9).

The majority of stent thromboses occurs early but may be observed even long time after PCI. Stent thrombosis often presents with STEMI, and emergency revascularization is indicated. Nonetheless, mortality (20–40%) and morbidity rates, including myocardial infarction (about 70%), are high.

Technical factors, including stent undersizing, incomplete stent apposition, residual stenosis or dissection, as well as pharmacological factors and particularly non-adherence to DAPT, are associated with acute thrombosis. Hence, after restoration of flow in the infarct-related artery, identification (possibly also by intracoronary imaging) of the underlying mechanism is warranted for proper treatment and avoidance of recurrence.

Table 2.8 Academic Research Consortium (ARC) classification of stent thrombosis

Definition	Definite:	Angiographic confirmation^
		Pathological confirmation#
	Probable:	Unexplained death ≤ 30 days
		Myocardial infarction related to ischaemia in the territory of implanted stent
	Possible:	Unexplained death > 30 days
Timing	Early:	Acute: 0–24
		Subacute: >24 h–30 days
	Late:	>30 days–1 year
	Very late:	>1 year

^ ≤48 h of acute onset of ischaemia at rest and/or new ischaemic electrocardiographic changes and/or typical rise and fall in biomarkers.

At autopsy or examination of material retrieved by thrombectomy.

As non-adherence to DAPT is largely the most important predictor of acute stent thrombosis, and given the poor prognosis of this complication, preventive measures, including ensuring compliance with DAPT, and optimal stent sizing and expansion are of paramount importance.

Although a true difference in the rate of stent thrombosis between BMS, and DES after 30 days from implantation is still debated, late and very late stent thromboses tend to occur more frequently with DES. Late and very late stent thrombosis require a more complex interplay among patient (diabetes, renal insufficiency, ACS, DAPT discontinuation), lesion (length, bifurcation, complex, vessel diameter), and procedural (number of stents, total stent length, use of DES, stent underexpansion, malapposition or fracture, residual thrombus or dissection) characteristics compared to acute thrombosis. Along with the same mechanical and pharmacological factors acting in acute stent thrombosis, additional mechanisms, including delayed endothelization, chronic inflammation (possibly due to hypersensitivity to polymer coating), and progression of atherosclerosis proximal or distal to the stent may be associated with late or very late stent thrombosis. Early discontinuation of DAPT however, still plays a predominant role.

Because the occurrence of stent thrombosis during DAPT with aspirin and clopidogrel may be related to non-responsiveness to clopidogrel, switching to a newer $P2Y_{12}$-receptor inhibitor (prasugrel or ticagrelor) may be considered in these cases. According to available data however, a strategy of $P2Y_{12}$-receptor inhibitor prescription based on laboratory tests of platelet inhibition is neither cost-effective nor recommended.

2.2.3 Restenosis (Table 2.9)

Following balloon angioplasty, several mechanisms, including migration and proliferation of smooth muscle cells, platelet deposition, thrombus formation, elastic recoil, and negative remodelling contribute to restenosis. As stent blocks elastic recoil and negative remodelling, the predominant mechanism for restenosis after stenting is neo-intimal hyperplasia. The incidence of restenosis varies according to the definition, either angiographic (>50% diameter stenosis at follow up angiography) or clinical (recurrence of angina and/or objective signs of ischaemia, and requiring target lesion/

Table 2.9 Post-procedural incidence of adverse events		
Adverse events	**Time period**	**(%)**
Combined death, myocardial infarction, stroke	1 year:	<1–4 in stable IHD ≥10 in ACS
Repeat revascularization §	1 year:	6–9
Restenosis	1 year:	30–40 (balloon angioplasty) 15–30 with BMS <10 with DES
Stent thrombosis	30 days:	<1
	1 year	1–2
	> 1 year	0.2–0.6 per year
Clinically relevant bleeding^	1 year	3–7

ACS = acute coronary syndrome; BMS = bare-metal stent; DES = drug-eluting stent; IHD = ischaemic heart disease
§ Target lesion/vessel.
^ Prompting evaluation and/or treatment, or fatal.

vessel revascularization), adopted. Less than 50% of patients with angiographic restenosis are symptomatic at one-year follow up, and 6% and 9% target lesion and vessel revascularizations, respectively, are generally performed at one year. Most patients with clinical restenosis present with recurrent exertional angina, but up to one-third may present with ACS (acute myocardial infarction in 5–10% and unstable angina in 25%).

Predictors of restenosis include the clinical setting in which PCI is performed (ACS), patient characteristics (diabetes, renal insufficiency, younger age, prior PCI, male gender, multivessel disease), lesion site (left main, ostial, saphenous vein graft), and procedural characteristics (stent size ≤2.5 mm, stent length ≥ 40 mm).

Treatment of restenosis depends on the initial PCI strategy, with stent (either BMS or DES) implantation being the recommended option after balloon angioplasty. Treatment of in-stent restenosis after BMS implantation includes balloon angioplasty, repeat BMS implantation, and DES implantation. Although balloon angioplasty may be an option in focal (<10 mm long) in-stent restenosis, in-stent implantation of DES is the preferred option for diffuse in-stent restenosis (>10 mm long, total occlusion). Angioplasty with paclitaxel-coated DEB may represent a better option compared to both balloon angioplasty and DES implantation for the treatment of restenosis following BMS implantation, owing to an observed reduction of MACE.

Owing to the increasing number of patients receiving DES, clinical in-stent restenosis after DES implantation is becoming increasingly common. In most cases, DES in-stent restenosis is focal. Resistance to anti-proliferative drugs, stent underexpansion, stent strut fracture, non-uniform stent strut coverage, gap in stent coverage, and residual noncovered atherosclerotic lesion may concur to the development of DES restenosis. Intracoronary imaging, either with intravascular ultrasound or optical coherence tomography, may be considered to determine the mechanism of restenosis and help guide proper treatment (balloon dilatation when previous stent is underexpanded, or repeat stenting when neo-intimal hyperplasia is predominant). Focal restenosis may be treated with balloon angioplasty, whereas more diffuse disease may be treated with either BMS, DES implantation with the same or an alternative anti-proliferative drug, or bypass surgery. Solid data regarding treatment with DEB of restenosis after DES implantation are yet unavailable. At present however, the most appropriate treatment of in-stent restenosis remains undetermined.

2.2.4 Adverse events (Table 2.9)

The overall occurrence of *adverse events*, including death, myocardial infarction, and stroke, as well as of *repeat revascularization*, greatly varies depending on whether PCI is performed in the context of stable IHD or ACS. Whereas most events are related to previous PCI (stent thrombosis, restenosis), progression of atherosclerosis in the native artery may also account for the recurrence of adverse cardiac events and the need for repeat revascularization. In contrast, bleeding is essentially attributable to the exposure of the patients to DAPT.

Bleeding is relatively frequent compared with ischaemic adverse events and has important prognostic and economic implications. In patients with ACS, whether or not undergoing PCI, bleeding is of particular prognostic relevance, as it is associated with higher mortality. Whereas individual factors, including advanced age, low body weight, female gender, chronic kidney disease, baseline anaemia, and especially previous gastrointestinal (GI) bleeding, are associated with the occurrence of bleeding, DAPT plays

Table 2.10 General recommendations to reduce the risk of bleeding during DAPT

Use of safest drugs
Lowest effective drug doses
Shortest possible duration of P2Y$_{12}$-receptor inhibitor
Routine gastric protection

DAPT = dual antiplatelet therapy

the major role, with an approximately 50% increase in risk when clopidogrel is added to aspirin. Such risk is further increased (by approximately 30%) when the newer P2Y$_{12}$-receptor inhibitors prasugrel and ticagrelor are used in place of clopidogrel.

During DAPT, most bleeding occurs in the GI tract, at a rate of about 2% per year. Because of that, routine gastric protection with proton-pump inhibitors (PPI) has been advocated. There is pharmacodynamic evidence that omeprazole (and esomeprazole) interferes with clopidogrel metabolism, thereby reducing its effect. Even though clear evidence that this laboratory finding has true clinical implications is lacking, concomitant use of PPI and DAPT is currently recommended only in patients at highest risk, such as those with prior GI bleeding. Such a strategy may also be considered in all patients in whom the risk of bleeding is deemed high (advanced age, concomitant use of oral anti-coagulants, nonsteroidal anti-inflammatory drugs, steroids, or *Helicobacter pylori* infection). When there is concern that the interaction between clopidogrel and omeprazole may put the patient at high risk of potentially catastrophic ischaemic events, either an alternative PPI which does not interfere with clopidogrel metabolism (pantoprazole) or use of the H$_2$-receptor antagonist ranitidine may be considered. Of note, the newer P2Y$_{12}$-receptor inhibitors prasugrel and ticagrelor have no interaction with PPI and therefore can be safely used in conjunction.

General measures to reduce the risk of bleeding during DAPT are summarized in Table 2.10.

The occurrence of bleeding in the post-procedural setting should generally be managed as in the peri-procedural period, and therefore not interrupting both antiplatelet agents (aspirin and P2Y$_{12}$-receptor inhibitor) at the same time, especially if the complication occurs within the period most vulnerable to stent thrombosis (one month for BMS, and 6–12 months for DES). After ≥6 months of DAPT have been completed following DES implantation, temporary withdrawal of one antiplatelet may be considered as relatively safe. Earlier (after ≥3 months) interruption of DAPT after DES implantation is likely safer when new-generation zotarolimus-, everolimus-, or polymer-free, amphilimus-DES have been used.

Key Reading

Agewall S, Cattaneo M, Collet JP, Andreotti F, Lip GY, Verheugt FW, Huber K, Grove EL, Morais J, Husted S, Wassmann S, Rosano G, Atar D, Pathak A, Kjeldsen K, Storey RF, on behalf of ESC Working Group on Cardiovascular Pharmacology and Drug Therapy and ESC Working Group on Thrombosis. Expert opinion paper on the use of proton pump inhibitors in patients with cardiovascular disease and antithrombotic therapy. *Eur Heart J* 2013; **34:** 1708–1713.

Buchanan GL, Basavarajaiah S, Chieffo A. Stent thrombosis: incidence, predictors and new technologies. *Thrombosis* 2012; **2012:** 956–62.

Byrne RA, Cassese S, Linhardt M, Kastrati A. Vascular access and closure in coronary angiography and percutaneous intervention. *Nat Rev Cardiol* 2013; **10:** 27–40.

Indermuehle A, Bahl R, Lansky AJ, Froehlich GM , Knapp G , Timmis A , Meier P. Drug-eluting balloon angioplasty for in-stent restenosis: a systematic review and meta-analysis of randomised controlled trials. *Heart* 2013; **99:** 327–33.

Kim BK, Hong MK, Shin DH, Nam CM, Kim JS, Ko YG, Choi D, Kang TS, Park BE, Kang WC, Lee SH, Yoon JH, Hong BK, Kwon HM, Jang Y; RESET Investigators. A new strategy for discontinuation of dual antiplatelet therapy: the RESET Trial (REal Safety and Efficacy of 3-month dual antiplatelet Therapy following Endeavor zotarolimus-eluting stent implantation). *J Am Coll Cardiol* 2012; **60:** 1340–8.

Kumbhani DJ, Bavry AA, Desai MY, Bangalore S, Bhatt DL. Role of aspiration and mechanical thrombectomy in patients with acute myocardial infarction undergoing primary angioplasty: an updated meta-analysis of randomized trials. *J Am Coll Cardiol* 2013; **62:** 1409–18.

Levine MN, Bates ER, Blankenship JC, Bailey SR, Bittl JA, Cercek B, Chambers CE, Ellis SG, Guyton RA, Hollenberg SM, Khot UN, Lange RA, Mauri L, Mehran R, Moussa ID, Mukherjee D, Nallamothu BK, Ting HH. 2011 ACCF/AHA/SCAI guideline for percutaneous coronary intervention: a report of the American College of Cardiology Foundation/American Heart Association Task Force on Practice Guidelines and the Society for Cardiovascular Angiography and Interventions. *Catheter Cardiovasc Interv* 2012; **79:** 453–95.

Sarno G, Lagerqvist B, Fröbert O, Nilsson J, Olivecrona G, Omerovic E, Saleh N, Venetzanos D, James S. Lower risk of stent thrombosis and restenosis with unrestricted use of "new-generation" drug-eluting stents: a report from the nationwide Swedish Coronary Angiography and Angioplasty Registry (SCAAR). *Eur Heart J* 2012; **33:** 606–13.

Steg PG, Huber K, Andreotti F, Arnesen H, Atar D, Badimon L, Bassand JP, De Caterina R, Eikelboom JA, Gulba D, Hamon M, Helft G, Fox KA, Kristensen SD, Rao SV, Verheugt FW, Widimsky P, Zeymer U, Collet JP. Bleeding in acute coronary syndromes and percutaneous coronary interventions: position paper by the Working Group on Thrombosis of the European Society of Cardiology. *Eur Heart J* 2011; **32:** 1854–64.

Chapter 3

Oral anticoagulation

Freek W. A. Verheugt, Sam Schulman, Andrea
Rubboli, Jonathan L. Halperin, Gregory Y. H. Lip

> ## Key points
> - Oral anticoagulation is indicated to prevent the occurrence and/or recurrence of arterial and venous thromboembolism.
> - Oral anticoagulation is a complex treatment requiring appropriate indications and careful management.
> - Vitamin K antagonists (warfarin, acenocoumarol, phenprocoumon), and newer, non-vitamin K antagonist direct inhibitors of thrombin (dabigatran) or of factor Xa (rivaroxaban, apixaban) are the oral anticoagulants currently available.
> - Bleeding is the most frequent unwanted effect of oral anticoagulation and may have important prognostic impact.
> - Stratification of the individual risk of thromboembolism and bleeding is advised prior to starting oral anticoagulation to optimize the risk-to-benefit ratio.

Oral anticoagulation (OAC) is the established mainstay for the prevention of the occurrence and/or recurrence of arterial and venous thromboembolism. By either inhibiting the hepatic synthesis of normally functioning vitamin K-dependent coagulation factors II (prothrombin), VII, IX, and X or directly blocking single coagulation factors IIa (thrombin) or Xa, OAC with vitamin K antagonists (VKA; warfarin, acenocoumarol, phenprocoumon) or newer, non-VKA, direct oral anticoagulants (NOAC; dabigatran, rivaroxaban, apixaban) aims at inducing a controlled and reversible depression of normal haemostatic mechanisms. Because of the delicate balance between haemostasis and anticoagulation, OAC is a complex therapy, so appropriate indications and careful management are required.

3.1 Indications

Based on the substantial risk of thromboembolism, OAC is warranted in the following three main clinical settings (Table 3.1): (non-valvular) atrial fibrillation (AF), prosthetic heart valve (PHV), and venous thromboembolism (VTE; deep vein thrombosis/pulmonary embolism). On average, OAC reduces the risk of thromboembolism by 65–80%.

Table 3.1 Average risk of thromboembolism without OAC

Clinical setting	(%)
AF	5/year
PHV	8/year
VTE	40 in the first month/10 during subsequent two months/3–10 up to one year

AF = atrial fibrillation; OAC = oral anticoagulation; PHV = prosthetic heart valve; VTE = venous thromboembolism

3.1.1 AF

The risk of stroke (or systemic embolism) is increased approximately five-fold by AF, which is similar in patients with either transient (paroxysmal/persistent) or permanent AF. AF is responsible for approximately 25% of all ischaemic strokes, and ischaemic strokes related to AF are generally more disabling and more often fatal than those of other aetiologies (secondary to cerebrovascular disease). Furthermore, the risk of stroke for patients who have already experienced a stroke or a transient ischaemic attack (TIA) is two and a half times greater than for patients who have not. Although on average 5%, the annual incidence of stroke in AF widely ranges between approximately 0% and 15%, depending on the presence and number of risk factors (left ventricle (LV) dysfunction, hypertension, advanced age, diabetes, prior cerebrovascular event, associated vascular disease, and female gender). Apart from patients with no risk factors or with female gender as the only risk factor, lifelong OAC is warranted in all patients with AF. Indeed, OAC with adjusted-dose VKA (warfarin in most cases) targeted to an International Normalized Ratio (INR) of 2.0–3.0 is highly effective in reducing the risk of stroke (Table 3.2).

Compared to adjusted-dose warfarin, NOAC have been shown to be comparably (dabigatran, 110 mg twice daily, and rivaroxaban, 20 mg once daily) or more (dabigatran, 150 mg twice daily, and apixaban, 5 mg twice daily) effective in stroke prevention (Table 3.2). Of note, only dabigatran, 150 mg twice daily, has been shown superior

Table 3.2 Relative reduction of the risk of stroke in AF

Regimen		(%)
Adjusted-dose warfarin	vs no treatment	64
	vs aspirin	38
	vs aspirin + clopidogrel	42
Dabigatran, 110/150 mg twice daily	vs adjusted-dose warfarin	9/34
Rivaroxaban, 20 mg once daily	vs adjusted-dose warfarin	12
Apixaban, 5 mg twice daily	vs adjusted-dose warfarin	21
	vs aspirin	55
Aspirin	vs no treatment	19
Aspirin + clopidogrel	vs aspirin	28

AF = atrial fibrillation

Table 3.3 Anticoagulation regimens in AF	
Dabigatran	110/150 mg twice daily
Rivaroxaban	20 mg once daily§
Apixaban	5 mg twice daily$^#$
VKA	individualized dose once daily (to maintain INR 2.0–3.0)

AF = atrial fibrillation; INR = International Normalized Ratio; VKA = vitamin K antagonists

§ To be reduced to 15 mg once daily when renal function impaired (creatinine clearance (CrCl) 15–49 ml/min).

$^#$ To be reduced to 2.5 mg twice daily when ≥2 of: age ≥80 years, weight ≤60 kg, and serum creatinine ≥1.5 ml/min.

to adjusted-dose warfarin for the prevention of ischaemic stroke. Favourable pharmacokinetics allowing for rapid onset and offset of effect, administration in fixed doses with no need for routine coagulation monitoring, the absence of food interaction, and the few drug interactions make NOAC more convenient. Because of that, as well as having comparable (dabigatran, 150 mg twice daily, and rivaroxaban, 20 mg once daily) or superior (dabigatran, 110 mg twice daily, and apixaban, 5 mg twice daily) safety to warfarin on major bleeding, and actually a superior safety on the incidence of intracranial bleeding (all three NOAC, at any dosage), NOAC are currently recommended as the first-line option for OAC in patients with AF (Table 3.3).

The role of antiplatelet therapy for stroke prevention in AF is very limited. Compared to no treatment, aspirin (and antiplatelet therapy in general) has little efficacy (Table 3.2), with no substantial benefit, especially in patients aged >75 years, on the occurrence of major bleeding and intracranial bleeding. Compared to apixaban, 5 mg twice daily, aspirin is less effective (Table 3.2), with no advantage on the occurrence of bleeding. Compared to dual antiplatelet therapy (DAPT) with aspirin and clopidogrel, aspirin is less effective (Table 3.2), although the risk of major bleeding is substantially less (approximately 40%). DAPT with aspirin and clopidogrel is less effective than adjusted-dose warfarin targeted to an INR of 2.0–3.0 (Table 3.2), with no difference in the occurrence of major bleeding.

At present, therefore, aspirin has no indication, either in patients at low risk (no risk factors), because of the very low incidence of stroke without antithrombotic therapy, or in those unsuitable for VKA in whom apixaban, 5 mg twice daily, has a superior efficacy-to-safety balance. DAPT with aspirin and clopidogrel is only indicated in patients who are not candidates for OAC for reasons other than increased risk of bleeding (unwillingness to take OAC or to undergo periodical monitoring). No data are available on DAPT with aspirin and a newer $P2Y_{12}$-receptor inhibitor (prasugrel, ticagrelor) for stroke prevention, and such combination is therefore currently not recommended. No solid evidence is available regarding non-pharmacological approaches to stroke prevention (left atrial appendage closure), which therefore are not generally recommended. Finally, a rhythm control strategy does not alter the burden of asymptomatic AF and thereby the indication for OAC.

3.1.2 PHV

The risk of stroke (or systemic embolism) is dependent on the type (mechanical vs biological), and site (mitral vs aortic) of PHV, as well as on the design (bileaflet vs tilting disc vs caged ball) and construction materials. Mechanical valves, mitral position, and older-design valves (caged ball or tilting disc) are associated with a greater risk of

Table 3.4 Antithrombotic therapy after heart valve treatment (with no risk factors for thromboembolism)

Heart valve treatment	Early (3 months)	Long-term
Aortic valve bioprosthesis	Aspirin	No treatment
Mitral (or tricuspid) valve bioprosthesis	VKA	Aspirin vs no treatment
Any mechanical valve prosthesis	VKA	VKA
Aortic or mitral surgical repair	Aspirin	No treatment
TAVI or percutaneous edge-to-edge mitral repair	DAPT	Aspirin

DAPT = dual antiplatelet therapy with aspirin and clopidogrel; TAVI = transcatheter aortic valve implantation; VKA = vitamin K antagonists

stroke. The recommended antithrombotic therapy for the various PHV types and positions, as well as valve interventions, is summarized in Table 3.4.

Administration of aspirin beyond the first three months after implantation of a biological PHV is not routinely recommended and should only be considered when other indications for antithrombotic treatment (atherosclerotic disease) are concomitant, or when the PHV has been implanted in the mitral position. Long-term, adjusted-dose VKA in patients with mechanical PHV reduces the risk of stroke by approximately 75%. Modern, bileaflet mechanical PHV are associated with a lower frequency of thromboembolic complications, which during effective OAC are estimated to be <1% and 3.5% per year in the aortic and mitral positions, respectively. Initial available evidence shows lower efficacy (as well as safety) of NOAC (dabigatran) compared to warfarin for stroke prevention in patients with PHV, and therefore NOAC must not be used in this setting.

The intensity (INR range) of OAC with adjusted-dose VKA should be established based on the estimated thrombogenicity of the mechanical PHV and the presence of additional risk factors for stroke (Table 3.5).

Addition of aspirin to VKA increases efficacy but at a cost, however, of increased risk of bleeding. Apart from when atherosclerotic disease is concomitant, this combination should only be considered after an episode of stroke, despite an INR within therapeutic range.

Table 3.5 INR range for mechanical PHV

Prosthesis thrombogenicity	No risk factors	≥1 risk factors*
Low	2.0–3.0	2.5–3.5
(Bileaflet valves: Carbomedics, Medtronic Hall, St. Jude Medical, ON-X)		
Medium	2.5–3.5	3.0–4.0
(Other bileaflet valves)		
High	3.0–4.0	3.5–4.5
(Lillehei-Kaster, Omniscience, Starr-Edwards, Björk-Shiley, other tilting disc valves)		

INR = International Normalized Ratio; PHV = prosthetic heart valve

* Mitral or tricuspid valve replacement, previous thromboembolism, atrial fibrillation, mitral stenosis of any degree, and left ventricle dysfunction (ejection fraction <35%).

3.1.3 VTE

Regardless of whether an episode of VTE is provoked by a reversible factor (immobilization, trauma, recent surgery) or it is unprovoked (idiopathic), the risk of recurrence is higher during the first three months and highest during the first month. Nonetheless, following the first three months, the risk of recurrence is higher when the index episode is unprovoked compared to provoked by reversible factors. Of note, deep vein thrombosis tends to recur as deep vein thrombosis, whereas pulmonary embolism, again as pulmonary embolism.

To minimize the risk of embolization of deep vein thrombosis, and therefore of pulmonary embolism, and to favour the dissolution of thrombi in the venous system in the legs and thromboemboli in the pulmonary circulation, early and effective anticoagulation is warranted upon recognition, and even suspicion, of VTE.

Traditional anticoagulation regimens include immediate administration of a parenteral anticoagulant, either intravenous (IV) unfractionated heparin (UFH) or subcutaneous (SC) low-molecular-weight heparin (LMWH) or fondaparinux, to be combined within the first or second day with VKA. Overlapping of the two treatments should continue for a minimum of five days, and the parenteral anticoagulant should be discontinued afterwards, provided that the INR is >2.0 for at least two consecutive days (Table 3.6).

Based on the comparable efficacy to conventional treatment with initial enoxaparin followed by adjusted-dose VKA on the recurrence of VTE, oral treatment with rivaroxaban may be considered from the beginning (Table 3.6). Owing to its favourable pharmacokinetics in fact, effective anticoagulation is rapidly (2–4 h) achieved after oral ingestion of a single dose of rivaroxaban.

OAC has been shown to reduce the risk of recurrence of VTE by approximately 80% and should therefore be continued beyond the early period. The optimal duration of OAC, however, is still controversial. In general, it is accepted that patients in whom the episode of VTE was provoked by a reversible factor should be treated for a shorter period than those with an unprovoked episode, persistent risk factors (cancer, thrombophilic state), or recurrent episodes (Table 3.7).

Of note, in patients with cancer, LMWH rather than adjusted-dose VKA should be prescribed for the first three to six months.

Extended treatment in patients with unprovoked VTE should not be intended as indefinite, but instead the decision to prolong OAC therapy beyond three months should include a careful evaluation of the balance of risks and benefits, and be periodically

Table 3.6 Anticoagulation regimens in VTE	
Immediate	IV UFH, 80 U/kg bolus + 18 U/kg/h infusion
	or SC enoxaparin, 1 mg/kg twice daily or 1.5 mg/kg once daily
	or SC fondaparinux, 5 mg (<50 kg BW), 7.5 mg (50–100 kg BW), 10 mg (>100 kg BW) once daily
	or PO rivaroxaban, 15 mg twice daily (for 3 weeks)
Extended	PO VKA (INR 2.0–3.0)
	or PO rivaroxaban, 20 mg once daily

BW = body weight; INR = International Normalized Ratio; IV = intravenous; PO = orally; SC = subcutaneous; UFH = unfractionated heparin; VKA = vitamin K antagonist

Table 3.7 Recommended duration of anticoagulation in VTE	
Provoked by reversible risk factor (immobilization, trauma, recent surgery)	3 months
Unprovoked	≥3 months*
Recurrent unprovoked	Indefinite

VTE = venous thromboembolism
* Extended anticoagulation to be considered when the International Normalized Ratio (INR) is stable and bleeding risk low.

reassessed. Additional variables, such as D-dimer levels, residual vein thrombosis, post-thrombotic syndrome, or right ventricular size and function, may be used to guide the decision to extend OAC in these patients. In patients with unprovoked VTE who have completed 6–18 months of OAC, a two-year course of low-dose (100 mg/day) aspirin may be considered to further reduce the risk of recurrence.

3.2 Management

3.2.1 Initiation

When initiating OAC with warfarin, the starting dose should be selected based on the clinical status of the patient (Table 3.8)

When starting with a 10 mg dose, an initial effect on the INR is apparent within two to three days, with a value ≥2.0 commonly reached after four to five days. Following the first two days of fixed-dose treatment, warfarin dosing should be arranged according to the INR value (Table 3.9).

INR monitoring is usually performed daily in hospitalized patients until the therapeutic range has been achieved and maintained for at least two consecutive days, and then two to three times weekly for one to two weeks, then less often depending on the stability of INR. In outpatients starting warfarin therapy, initial monitoring may be reduced to every few days until a stable INR has been obtained.

When NOAC are used in patients with AF (and VTE for rivaroxaban only), the standard, fixed dose of each drug should be given (Tables 3.3, 3.6), with the anticoagulant effect expected to appear within a few (two to four) hours. No loading dose or laboratory monitoring is required. However, careful selection of the appropriate dose should be carried out based on: a) renal function, as these drugs are to a various degree all cleared by the kidney, and are contraindicated in the presence of severe renal failure (creatinine clearance (CrCl) <15–30 ml/min), and b) haemorrhagic risk, which in turn is related to age, renal function, body weight, co-morbidities, and co-medications (Table 3.10).

3.2.2 Maintenance

In OAC with adjusted-dose VKA, the efficacy (prevention of thromboembolism) and safety (avoidance of bleeding complications) is dependent on the time the INR

Table 3.8 Warfarin dosing for the first two days of treatment	
'Healthy' (suitable for outpatient management) patients	10 mg/day
Hospitalized patients	5 mg/day
Sick (liver disease, congestive heart failure) or elderly patients	≤5 mg/day

Table 3.9	Warfarin dosing to achieve INR of 2.0–3.0 after the first two days	
	INR value	**Dose to be given**
Day 3	<1.5	1–1½× initial dose
	1.5–1.9	Continue initial dose
	2.0–2.5	½–1× initial dose
	2.6–3.0	½× initial dose
	>3.0	Hold dose
Day 4	<1.5	1½–2× initial dose
	1.5–1.9	1–1½× initial dose
	2.0–2.5	Continue last dose
	2.6–2.9	¾× initial dose
	3.0–3.5	Hold dose
	>3.5	Hold dose
Day 5	<1.5	2× initial dose
	1.5–1.9	1½–2× initial dose
	2.0–2.5	Continue last dose
	2.6–2.9	¾× initial dose
	3.0–3.5	½× initial dose
	>3.5	Hold dose
Day 6	<1.5	2× initial dose
	1.5–1.9	1½–2× initial dose
	2.0–2.5	Continue last dose
	2.6–2.9	Continue last dose
	3.0–3.5	¾× initial dose
	>3.5	Hold dose
Day 7	<2.0	2× initial dose
	2.0–2.5	Continue last dose
	2.6–2.9	Continue last dose
	3.0–3.5	¾× initial dose
	>3.5	¾× initial dose

is maintained within the therapeutic range. Although in common practice the time in therapeutic range (TTR) is only about 50–55%, careful monitoring of OAC should be arranged aiming at a TTR ≥70%. Computerized algorithms and patient self-management have been shown to improve warfarin dose adjustments, and to increase the TTR. At present, high-quality anticoagulation management delivered by an anticoagulation clinic is an accepted and effective method for managing OAC.

INR testing following initiation of OAC can be gradually reduced to intervals as long as every four weeks, or even every 12 weeks in patients with consistently stable INR.

Table 3.10 Initial (and maintenance) dose of NOAC for AF

	Dabigatran	Rivaroxaban	Apixaban
Standard patient	150 mg twice daily	20 mg once daily	5 mg twice daily
Moderate renal failure (CrCL 30–49 ml/min)	150 mg twice daily	15 mg once daily	5 mg twice daily
Advanced age (≥75–80 years)	110 mg twice daily	20 mg once daily	5 mg twice daily
High haemorrhagic risk*	110 mg twice daily	15 mg once daily	2.5 mg twice daily

AF = atrial fibrillation; CrCl = creatinine clearance; NOAC = newer, non-vitamin K antagonist, direct oral anticoagulants
* Combination of advanced age, low body weight, concomitant antiplatelets, impaired renal function.

If dose adjustments are required, the cycle of more frequent monitoring is repeated until a stable response is again obtained (Table 3.11).

Whereas temporary (≤5–7 days) INR values below the therapeutic range do not substantially increase the risk of thromboembolism, the risk of bleeding increases when INR is >4.0 and sharply increases with values >4.5. Periodical INR monitoring allows the detection of supratherapeutic values so that they may be corrected accordingly (Table 3.11).

As opposed to VKA, NOAC do not require routine laboratory monitoring for assessment of OAC intensity. Yet, periodical (every 6–12 months) clinical and laboratory (complete blood count (CBC), CrCl) monitoring is warranted to assess compliance, evaluate side effects and complications, detect co-medications, and check renal function.

3.2.3 Bleeding

The incidence of bleeding during OAC with adjusted-dose VKA is variable and depends on the definition and classification of bleeding, design of the studies, and patient population (Table 3.12).

Table 3.11 Warfarin dosing to achieve INR of 2.0–3.0 after the first week

INR < 1.5	Consider booster dose at 1½–2× daily maintenance dose Consider resumption of prior maintenance dose, if INR decrease is due to transient factors Increase weekly dose by 10–20%
INR 1.5–1.9	Consider booster dose at 1½–2× daily maintenance dose Consider resumption of prior maintenance dose, if INR decrease is due to transient factors Increase weekly dose by 5–15%
INR 2.0–3.3	Continue current dose
INR 3.4–4.0	Consider holding 1 dose Consider resumption of prior maintenance dose, if INR increase is due to transient factors Decrease weekly dose by 5–15%
INR 4.1–5.0	Hold 1–2 doses AND decrease weekly dose by 10–20%
INR 5.1–9.0	Hold 3 doses AND decrease weekly dose by 15–20% Consider vitamin K, 1–2.5 mg PO if concerned about bleeding
INR >9.0	Hold warfarin AND give vitamin K PO 2.5–5.0 mg Restart warfarin when INR reaches 2.0–3.0 AND decrease weekly dose by 15–20%

PO = orally; INR = International Normalized Ratio

Table 3.12 Average incidence/year of bleeding during long-term OAC with adjusted-dose VKA

Incidence of bleeding	(%)
Overall	10.0–17.0
Major	2.0–5.0
Fatal	0.5–1.0
Intracranial	0.2–0.4

OAC = oral anticoagulation; VKA = vitamin K antagonist

Among all bleeding complications, intracranial bleeding is the most feared because of its high disability and fatality rate.

During extended treatment with NOAC in AF, the incidence of major bleeding is comparable to warfarin for dabigatran, 150 mg twice daily, and rivaroxaban, 20 mg once daily, and significantly lower (by approximately 20–30%) with dabigatran, 110 mg twice daily, and apixaban, 5 mg twice daily. All NOAC at any dosage significantly and markedly (by approximately 30–70%) reduce the occurrence of intracranial bleeding. When used in VTE, rivaroxaban, 15 mg, twice daily for three weeks followed by 20 mg once daily is associated with an incidence of major bleeding comparable to the standard treatment of enoxaparin followed by adjusted-dose warfarin.

The occurrence of bleeding during OAC has relevant prognostic and management implications. Major bleeding may be life-threatening when occurring at critical sites (head, pericardium, pleura) or when leading to shock. Furthermore, major bleeding complications are generally associated with OAC discontinuation, which in turn contributes to adverse outcomes by leaving the patient exposed to an increased risk of thromboembolism. Because the case-fatality rate of major bleeding during OAC may be as high as 10%, identification of patients at risk, prevention of bleeding, and prompt and effective treatment when it occurs are of paramount importance. Numerous factors, including individual characteristics, intensity, timing and quality of OAC, and use of concomitant medications, have been established to impact on the risk of bleeding (Table 3.13).

Table 3.13 Factors associated with increased risk of bleeding during OAC

Age >65–70 years
Female gender
Genetics (CYP2C9 and/or VKORC1 gene polymorphism)*
Higher intensity of anticoagulation (INR >4.5* or higher dosage of NOAC)
Labile INR (TTR <60%)*
First 90 days of anticoagulation*
History of bleeding
Co-morbidities (hypertension, heart failure, malignancy, liver and/or renal disease, anaemia)
Co-medications (antiplatelet drugs, non-steroidal anti-inflammatory drugs)

CYP = cytochrome P450; INR = International Normalized Ratio; NOAC = newer, non-vitamin K, direct oral anticoagulants; OAC = oral anticoagulation; TTR = time in therapeutic range; VKORC1 = vitamin K epoxide reductase subunit 1
* With VKA.

Elderly patients have a more than two-fold higher risk of overall bleeding and intracranial bleeding compared to younger patients. Genetic factors, including polymorphism of genes encoding for enzymes involved in VKA metabolism, such as cytochrome P450 (CYP) 2C9, and vitamin K epoxide reductase subunit 1 (VKORC1) may also affect the response to warfarin and the stabilization of INR. So far, however, there is no evidence that pharmacogenetic dosing reduces the risk for bleeding. The most important risk factors for haemorrhage in patients on OAC with adjusted-dose VKA are the intensity and quality of OAC. INR values >4.5 are associated with an exponential increase in the risk of bleeding, whereas INR values <2.5 are associated with a two-fold increase in the risk of death for one unit. With respect to the quality of OAC with adjusted-dose VKA, a TTR below 60% is associated with an increased risk of both thromboembolism and major bleeding compared to TTR above 75%. Both as a marker of increased patient frailty and a cause of concomitant use of other medications, co-morbidities including hypertension, heart or renal failure, malignancy, and anaemia substantially increase the risk of haemorrhagic complications. Of note, the presence and degree of renal failure is of paramount importance as a risk factor for haemorrhagic complications in patients treated with NOAC because of their common elimination, albeit at different degrees, by the renal route. Hence, in the presence of renal failure, the plasma concentration of the drug may increase and thereby also the risk of bleeding. Finally, concomitant use of other antithrombotic agents, such as aspirin, and clopidogrel (or other $P2Y_{12}$–receptor inhibitors), alone or in combination, or non-steroidal anti-inflammatory drugs, is another predictor of bleeding, especially in the elderly where these drugs are commonly used.

3.2.4 Management of bleeding

In the event that bleeding occurs, the management is mainly driven by its severity. Mild and/or local bleeding may be managed only by holding one or more doses of the anticoagulant drug (either VKA or NOAC), associated with local compression. A more rapid reversal of anticoagulation (approximately 12–24 h when renal function is normal) is expected with NOAC compared to warfarin, owing to their much shorter half-life. Major or life-threatening bleeding requires a more complex management (Figure 3.1). Of note, no established antidote is currently available for any of the NOAC.

Whereas INR provides a rapid assessment of the effect of VKA, the absence of a ready-to-use and reliable laboratory test for the measurement of the activity of NOAC adds complexity to the management of bleeding. In case of emergency or severe bleeding, the activated partial prothrombin time (aPTT) or thrombin time for dabigatran and the prothrombin time (PT; using a reagent sensitive to the drug) for rivaroxaban may be used to estimate the presence of effective anticoagulation but not to quantify it. A quantitative assessment of the effect of dabigatran may be obtained with a specifically calibrated (Hemoclot) diluted thrombin time. No test is currently suggested for apixaban, but plasma levels can be measured by anti-factor Xa assays. Normal values for aPTT and/or thrombin time, and PT, as well as normal anti-Xa activity suggest that no clinically relevant anticoagulation effect of dabigatran, rivaroxaban, and apixaban is present.

Following treatment of a complication, OAC should then be restarted, but not earlier than 24 h after effective and definitive control of bleeding. Of note, restarting OAC with VKA will achieve effective anticoagulation only after several days, whereas the administration of NOAC will generate effective anticoagulation in a few (two to four) hours.

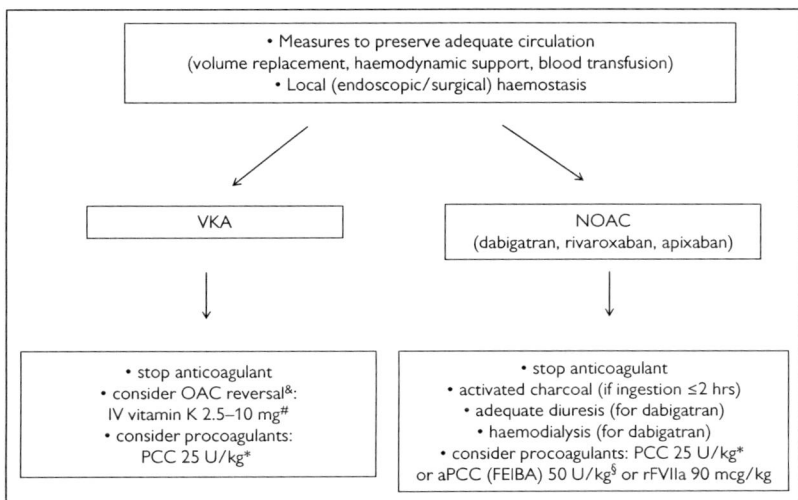

Figure 3.1 Management strategies for severe and/or life-threatening bleeding during OAC.

PCC = prothrombin complex concentrates; aPCC = activated prothrombin complex concentrates; FEIBA = Factor Eight Inhibitor Bypassing Activity; rFVIIa = recombinant factor VIIa; & reversal of anticoagulation expected ≥24 h; # 2.5–5.0 mg for INR <7, 5.0-10.0 mg for INR >7; * to be given once or twice; § maximum daily dose 200 U/kg

3.2.5 Peri-operative/intervention

In patients on OAC needing surgery or intervention (coronary angiography, arrhythmia catheter ablation, implantation of pacemaker or cardioverter-defibrillator), the decision to continue or interrupt OAC (with or without bridging with parenteral anticoagulants) is dictated by the balance between: a) risk of thromboembolism due to the condition for which OAC is indicated (Table 3.1), and b) risk of bleeding due to the surgical/invasive procedure. For most surgical interventions, withdrawal of OAC is required. OAC with warfarin should be interrupted five days before (last dose six days before), whereas the interruption should be between 24 h and four to five days when NOAC are used, depending on the drug, the patient's renal function, and the risk of bleeding from surgery (Table 3.14).

Whereas the short interruption of OAC required with NOAC (owing to the short half-life, correspondent rapid offset, and subsequent onset of action) generally does not mandate bridging anticoagulation with parenteral anticoagulants, in patients at moderate or high risk of thromboembolism (Table 3.15) in whom VKA have been interrupted, bridging anticoagulation with SC LMWH (enoxaparin) at therapeutic doses should be considered or implemented (Table 3.16).

The first dose of enoxaparin should be given two days after stopping warfarin (three days before surgery/intervention), when generally the INR has fallen <2.0, and the last dose, 24 h before intervention. Following surgery/intervention, warfarin can be reinitiated within 24 h, whereas enoxaparin and NOAC should be restarted not earlier than between 24 and 48 to 72 hours from standard and high bleeding risk surgery respectively, provided that adequate haemostasis has been achieved.

Albeit classified as minor procedures, colonoscopic polypectomy and biopsy of prostate or kidney carry an increased risk of bleeding, and the management should be similar to general surgery. In contrast, minor procedures like tooth extractions or endodontic procedures, small skin excisions, and cataract removal do not require interruption of OAC with warfarin, provided that optimal local haemostasis (possibly also using agents like tranexamic acid, 500 mg, five to ten minutes before and three to four times daily for the next one to two days) is obtained. Owing to the more convenient management of NOAC, temporary (one to two days) interruption of these drugs is probably preferable even for minor procedures. Alternatively, procedures at low bleeding risk and allowing adequate local haemostasis may be performed at trough level of plasma concentration (approximately 12 and 24 h from the last intake of dabigatran or apixaban, and rivaroxaban respectively), with no NOAC interruption.

In patients on warfarin undergoing arrhythmia catheter ablation or implantation of a cardioverter-defibrillator, OAC may be continued throughout the procedure because such an approach appears at least as safe and effective as warfarin interruption plus either SC LMWH or IV UFH. Furthermore, the uninterrupted approach significantly decreases in-hospital stay and costs. On the other hand, because of the rapid offset and subsequent onset of action and the lack of consistent data with uninterrupted treatment, NOAC should be temporarily interrupted before procedure (one to four or five days, depending on the drug used and the patient's renal function) without bridging anticoagulation (Table 3.14), and subsequently (after 24–48 h) reinitiated. For patients undergoing arrhythmia catheter ablation, both during uninterrupted warfarin treatment or interruption of OAC with either warfarin or NOAC, intra-procedural anticoagulation with IV UFH should be carried out according to standard regimen (50–100 U/kg bolus followed by 1000–1500 U/h infusion to achieve an activated clotting time ≥300 s).

3.3 Thromboembolism, and bleeding risk stratification

Because of the delicate balance between anticoagulation and haemostasis, the indication for OAC, as well as its management, should be based upon the absolute risks of

Table 3.14 NOAC interruption based on renal function and bleeding risk of surgery					
Creatinine clearance		Standard bleeding risk*: (stop 2–3 half-lives before)		High bleeding risk#: (stop 4–5 half-lives before)	
		last dose	doses to skip	last dose	doses to skip
>50 ml/min	dabigatran	2 days before	2	3 days before	4
	rivaroxaban	2 days before	1	3 days before	2
	apixaban	2 days before	2	3 days before	4
30–50 ml/min	dabigatran	3 days before	4	4–5 days before	6–8
	rivaroxaban	2 days before	1	3 days before	2
	apixaban	3 days before	4	4 days before	6

NOAC = newer, non-vitamin K antagonist, direct oral anticoagulants

* 2-day risk of major bleed: 0–2%.

2-day risk of major bleed: 2–4%.

Table 3.15 Peri-operative/intervention stratification of the risk of thromboembolism

Category	Absolute risk	AF	PHV	VTE
High	ATE >10% per yr	CHA$_2$DS$_2$-VASc score ≥5	Any mechanical mitral valve	Recent (<3 mos.) VTE
	VTE >10% per mo.	Recent (<3 mos.) stroke/TIA	Older aortic mechanical valve*	Severe thrombophilia §
		Rheumatic VHD	Recent (<6 mos.) stroke/TIA	
Moderate	ATE 4–10% per yr	CHA$_2$DS$_2$-VASc score 4–5	Bileaflet aortic mechanical valve+	VTE within past 3–12 mos.
	VTE 4–10% per mo.		≥1 risk factor$^#$	Non-severe thrombophilia$^∧$
			Bileaflet aortic mechanical valve	Recurrent VTE
			Without any risk factors$^#$	Active cancer
Low	ATE <4% per yr	CHA$_2$DS$_2$-VASc score 0–3	—	VTE >12 mos.
	VTE <4% per mo.			

AF = atrial fibrillation; ATE = arterial thromboembolism; CHA$_2$DS$_2$-VASc = **C**ongestive heart failure, **H**ypertension, **A**ge ≥75 years, **D**iabetes, prior **S**troke/transient ischaemic attack/systemic embolism, associated **V**ascular disease, **A**ge 65–74 years, and female **S**ex category; mo. = month; PHV = prosthetic heart valve; TIA = transient ischaemic attack; VHD = valvular heart disease; VTE = venous thromboembolism; yr = year

* Caged ball, tilting disc.

§ Deficiency of protein C, protein S, or antithrombin; antiphospholipid syndrome; multiple abnormalities.

$^#$ Atrial fibrillation, heart failure, hypertension, age ≥75 years, diabetes, stroke/TIA.

$^∧$ Heterozygous factor V or factor II mutation.

thromboembolism and bleeding, as well as the anticipated net clinical benefit for the individual patient.

3.3.1 Thromboembolism risk stratification

Among and within the three main clinical settings warranting OAC, namely AF, PHV, and VTE, the risk of thromboembolism is not homogeneous.

In patients with AF, the incidence of stroke (or systemic embolism) is related to major and clinically relevant non-major risk factors (Table 3.17).

Table 3.16 Suggested peri-operative/intervention management of OAC with VKA

Thromboembolic risk	Strategy	Regimen
High	Bridging	SC enoxaparin 0.8–1.0 mg/kg twice daily
Moderate	Bridging vs no bridging$^#$	SC enoxaparin 0.8–1.0 mg/kg twice daily vs none
Low	No bridging	None

OAC = oral anticoagulation; SC = subcutaneous; VKA = vitamin K antagonists

$^#$ To be decided based on assessment of individual patient- and surgery-related factors.

Table 3.17 Risk factors for stroke in AF

Major	Previous stroke/TIA/systemic embolism
	Age ≥75 years
Clinically relevant non-major	Heart failure or moderate/severe LV dysfunction*
	Hypertension
	Diabetes
	Female gender
	Age 65–74 years
	Vascular disease #

LV = left ventricle; TIA = transient ischaemic attack

* LV ejection fraction ≤40%.

\# Prior myocardial infarction, peripheral artery disease, aortic plaque.

Based on the presence, and number of risk factors, an assessment of the stroke risk can be performed and the indication for OAC established in accordance (Figure 3.2).

The risk factor-based approach can be expressed as CHA_2DS_2-VASc (**C**ongestive heart failure, **H**ypertension, **A**ge ≥75 years, **D**iabetes, previous **S**troke/TIA/systemic

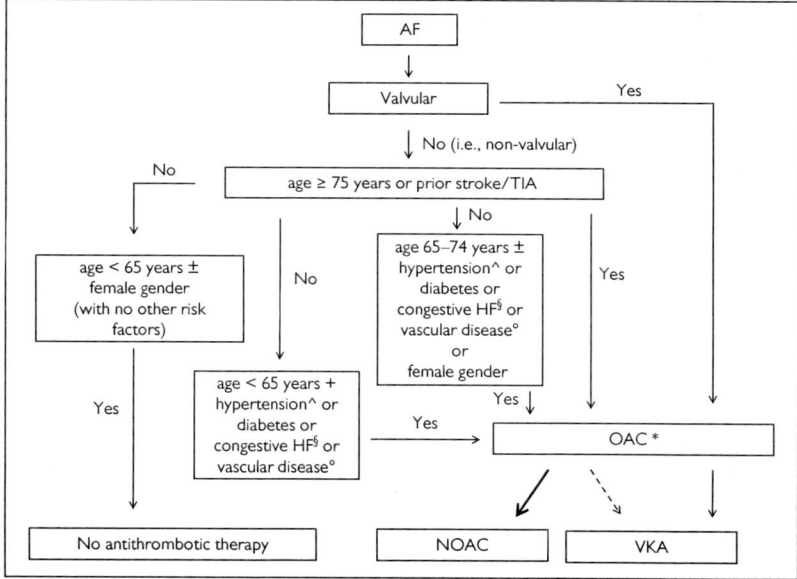

Figure 3.2 Indications for antithrombotic therapy in AF according to the risk of stroke.

AF = atrial fibrillation; HF = heart failure; NOAC = newer, non-vitamin K, direct oral anticoagulants; OAC= oral anticoagulation; TIA = transient ischaemic attack; VKA = vitamin K antagonist; * bleeding risk assessment warranted before initiating OAC; ^ uncontrolled hypertension; § New York Heart Association (NYHA) class II and/or left ventricle ejection fraction ≤40%; ° prior myocardial infarction, peripheral artery disease, aortic plaque.

Table 3.18 Risk of stroke in AF patients according to CHA_2DS_2-VASc score

CHA_2DS_2-VASc score	0	1	2	3	4	5	6	7	8	9
Incidence/year (%)	0	1.3	2.2	3.2	4.0	6.7	9.8	9.6	6.7	15.2

AF = atrial fibrillation

embolism, associated **V**ascular disease, **A**ge 65–74 years, female **S**ex category) score, where 2 points each are assigned to age ≥75 years and previous stroke/TIA/systemic embolism, and 1 point each to congestive heart failure/LV dysfunction, history of hypertension, diabetes, age 65–74 years, associated vascular disease, and female gender. Of note, female gender is not an independent predictor for increased stroke risk but would be relevant in patients aged ≥65 when present in addition to other stroke risk factors.

The risk of stroke is additive and progressively increases as the risk factors add up (Table 3.18).

In patients with at least one major or two clinically relevant, non-major risk factors (CHA_2DS_2-VASc score ≥2), but also in those with only one clinically relevant, non-major risk factor (CHA_2DS_2-VASc score 1), not including however female gender, OAC with NOAC, or alternatively with VKA, is warranted, owing to the favourable benefit to risk ratio (risk/year of major bleeding with OAC 1–2% vs risk/year of stroke without OAC 2–15%).

In patients with *PHV*, the stratification of the risk of thromboembolism is essentially based on the type of prosthesis (mechanical vs biological), with the position (mitral vs tricuspid vs aortic) helping in further refining risk assessment (Figure 3.3).

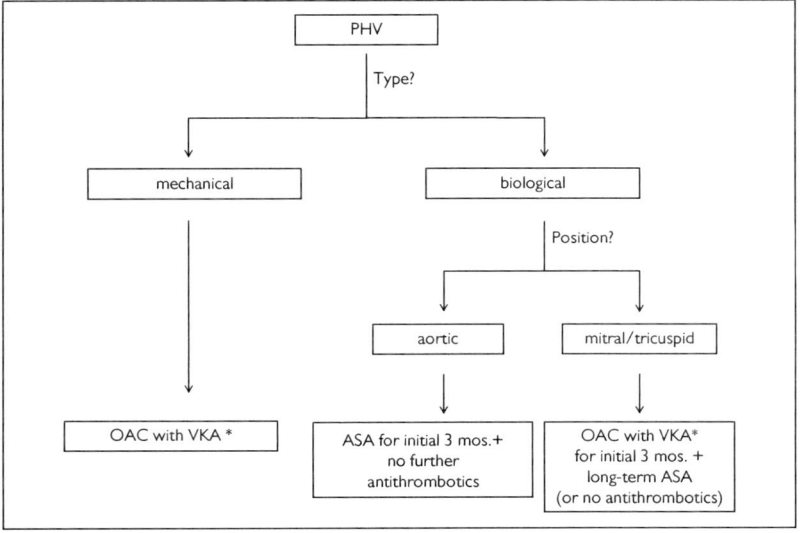

Figure 3.3 Indications for antithrombotic therapy in PHV according to the risk of stroke.

ASA = aspirin; mos. = months; OAC = oral anticoagulation; PHV = prosthetic heart valve; VKA = vitamin K antagonist; * bleeding risk assessment warranted before initiating OAC.

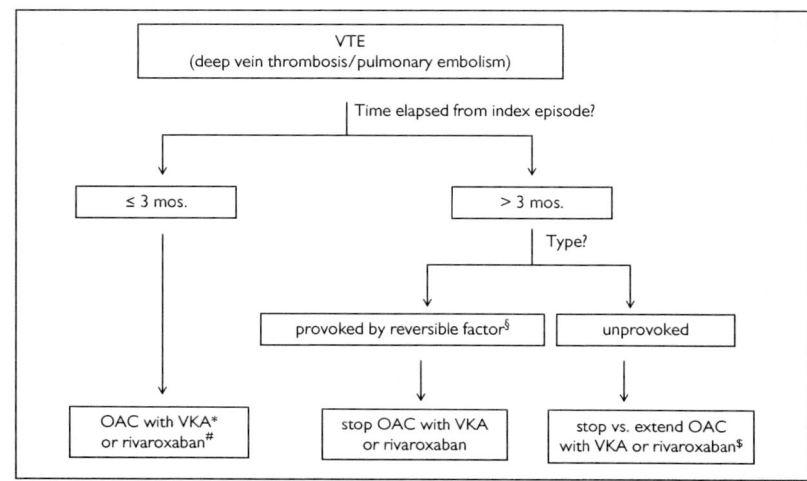

Figure 3.4 Indication for antithrombotic therapy in VTE according to the risk of occurrence/recurrence.
OAC = oral anticoagulation; VKA = vitamin K antagonist; VTE = venous thromboembolism; § immobilization, trauma, recent surgery; * to be overlapped at onset with LMWH, or fondaparinux; # bleeding risk assessment warranted before initiating OAC; $ decision to continue long-term OAC to be taken based on careful assessment of risk/benefit ratio.

As previously mentioned, in patients with mechanical PHV, an increased intensity of OAC (higher INR range) may be advised when additional risk factors for stroke (AF, previous stroke/systemic embolism, LV dysfunction) are present.

In patients with VTE, the stratification of the risk of occurrence/recurrence is essentially based on the time elapsed from (≤3 vs >3 months), and the type (provoked by a reversible factor vs unprovoked) of the index episode (Figure 3.4).

3.3.2 Bleeding risk stratification

Because bleeding is the major and most frequent side effect of OAC and has a relevant prognostic impact, the risk of bleeding should be assessed together with the risk of thromboembolism prior to starting OAC. Bleeding risk stratification is more complex, and many risk factors for bleeding are also risk factors for stroke.

Various schemes have been developed to identify patients at higher risk of major bleeding during OAC with VKA. Among them, the HAS-BLED (**H**ypertension, **A**bnormal liver or kidney function, prior **S**troke, **B**leeding history or predisposition, **L**abile INR, **E**lderly, and concomitant **D**rugs) score is the simplest (Table 3.19), and the one which performs best. Please note, however, that the absolute predictive ability of the HAS-BLED score is modest.

Albeit derived from and initially validated in AF patients on OAC with VKA, the HAS-BLED score has been shown to perform well also in non-AF patients, and for antithrombotic therapies other than VKA (NOAC, antiplatelets). The HAS-BLED score retains its value in predicting intracranial bleeding, as well as major extracranial bleeding.

Table 3.19 HAS-BLED (*H*ypertension, *A*bnormal liver or kidney function, prior *S*troke, *B*leeding history or predisposition, *L*abile INR, *E*lderly, and concomitant *D*rugs) score*

	Points
Hypertension**	1
Abnormal liver§ or kidney function^ (1 point each)	1 or 2
Stroke	1
Bleeding history or predisposition°	1
Labile INR$	1
Elderly (≥65 years)	1
Drugs #, or alcohol (1 point each)	1 or 2

INR = International Normalized Ratio

* Associated risk of major bleeding as determined by number of points: Low (<1%/year) = 0 points; Moderate (3–4%/year) = 1–2 points; High (5–9%/year) ≥3 points.

** Systolic blood pressure >160 mmHg.

§ Chronic hepatic disease (cirrhosis), or biochemical evidence of significant hepatic derangement (bilirubin >2× upper normal limit, or transaminase >3× upper normal limit).

^ Chronic dialysis, or renal transplantation, or creatinine >200 micromol/l.

° Bleeding diathesis, anaemia.

$ Unstable/high INR or time in therapeutic range (TTR) <60%.

Antiplatelets or non-steroidal anti-inflammatory drugs.

A HAS-BLED score ≥3 indicates high risk for major bleeding, thereby warranting some caution and regular review in order to assess whether modifiable risk factors (high blood pressure, labile INR, concomitant antiplatelets or non-steroidal anti-inflammatory drugs) have been corrected and the bleeding risk changed in accordance. A high HAS-BLED score should not be used on its own to exclude patients from OAC because whenever OAC is indicated (moderate-high risk of thromboembolism), a net clinical benefit of this treatment is observed, regardless of the initial risk of bleeding.

Key Reading

Eikelboom JW, Connolly SJ, Brueckmann M, Granger CB, Kappetein AP, Mack MJ, Blatchford J, Devenny K, Friedman J, Guiver K, Harper R, Khder Y, Lobmeyer MT, Maas H, Voigt JW, Simoons ML, Van de Werf F, for the RE-ALIGN Investigators. Dabigatran versus warfarin in patients with mechanical heart valves. *N Engl J Med* 2013; **369:** 1206–14.

Heidbuchel H, Verhamme P, Alings M, Antz M, Hacke W, Oldgren J, Sinnaeve P, Camm AJ, Kirchof P. European Heart Rhythm Association Practical Guide on the use of new oral anticoagulants in patients with non-valvular atrial fibrillation. *Europace* 2013; **15:** 625–51.

Lip GY, Andreotti F, Fauchier L, Huber K, Hylek E, Knight E, Levi M, Marin F, Palareti G, Kirchof P. Bleeding risk assessment and management in atrial fibrillation patients: a position document from the European Heart Rhythm Association, endorsed by the European Society of Cardiology Working Group on Thrombosis. *Eur Heart J* 2011; **13:** 723–46.

Lip GY. Stroke and bleeding risk assessment in atrial fibrillation: when, how, and why? *Eur Heart J* 2013; **34:** 1041–9.

Peacock WF, Gearhart MM, Mills RM. Emergency management of bleeding associated with old and new oral anticoagulants. *Clin Cardiol* 2012; **35:** 730–7.

Schulman S. Advances in the management of venous thromboembolism. *Best Pract Clin Haematol* 2012; **25:** 361–77.

Siegal D, Yudin J, Kaatz S, Douketis JD, Lim W, Spyropoulos AC. Periprocedural heparin bridging in patients receiving vitamin K antagonists: systematic review and meta-analysis of bleeding and thromboembolic rates. *Circulation* 2012; **126:** 1630–9.

Spyropoulos AC, Douketis JD. How I treat anticoagulated patients undergoing an elective procedure or surgery. *Blood* 2012; **120:** 2954–62.

Chapter 4

Percutaneous coronary intervention in the patient on oral anticoagulation

K. E. Juhani Airaksinen, Andrea Rubboli, Deepak L. Bhatt, Eric Eeckhout, Gregory Y. H. Lip

---

Key points

- Owing to the need to balance the risk of thromboembolism, stent thrombosis, major adverse cardiac events, and bleeding, the management of antithrombotic therapy in patients on oral anticoagulation undergoing percutaneous coronary intervention is complex.
- To minimize the risk of peri-procedural bleeding, extensive use of radial approach, avoidance of glycoprotein IIb/IIIa inhibitors, and uninterrupted oral anticoagulation with vitamin K antagonists are advised.
- Triple therapy with vitamin K antagonist, aspirin, and clopidogrel is the standard antithrombotic regimen throughout the period vulnerable to stent thrombosis.
- Because of the increased risk of bleeding, triple therapy of vitamin K antagonist, aspirin, and clopidogrel should be maintained for the least amount of time possible and managed with special care.
- Owing to the paucity of data regarding newer, more potent antiplatelet agents and newer, non-vitamin K antagonist, direct oral anticoagulants, the role of these agents is currently uncertain.

Although several peri- and post-procedural issues need to be addressed and meticulously cared for to balance the risks of major adverse cardiac events (MACE; death, myocardial infarction, need for repeat revascularization), stent thrombosis, and bleeding of percutaneous coronary intervention (PCI) with stent implantation in the ordinary patient, greater attention and care is required for the patient on oral anticoagulation (OAC). Because of the increased risk of thromboembolism of the condition requiring OAC, including (non-valvular) atrial fibrillation (AF), prosthetic heart valve (PHV), and venous thromboembolism (VTE), the increased risk of bleeding associated with PCI performed during uninterrupted OAC and with combined OAC and antiplatelet therapy following the procedure needs to be carefully weighed against the increased risk of thromboembolism

39

associated with the (even temporary) withdrawal of OAC and the risk of stent thrombosis associated with abstention from dual antiplatelet therapy (DAPT).

4.1 Peri-procedural issues

4.1.1 Anticoagulation (Tables 4.1, 4.2)

Similarly to ordinary patients and those patients on long-term OAC with either vitamin K antagonists (VKA) or newer, non-VKA, direct oral anticoagulants (NOAC; dabigatran, rivaroxaban, apixaban), effective intra-procedural anticoagulation is required during PCI to prevent the formation of thrombus on the intravascular instrumentarium and minimize thrombus formation at the site of balloon-induced plaque rupture.

As OAC patients are already anticoagulated, it should be decided, whenever PCI is non-emergency, whether to: a) continue OAC throughout PCI, or b) interrupt OAC prior to PCI, with or without bridging with intravenous (IV) unfractionated heparin (UFH) or subcutaneous (SC) low-molecular-weight heparin (LMWH), namely enoxaparin.

In patients on OAC with VKA, the uninterrupted strategy should be preferred. Warfarin, in fact, is capable of prolonging the activated clotting time (ACT) in a predictable fashion, and therapeutic (International Normalized Ratio (INR) ≥2.0), uninterrupted OAC with warfarin is not associated with increased peri-procedural thromboembolic or bleeding complications in patients undergoing PCI (nor in those undergoing elective surgery or invasive procedures, including arrhythmia catheter ablation, and implantation of pacemaker or cardioverter-defibrillator), in whom, on the contrary, the incidence of thromboembolic complications may even be increased by temporary under-therapeutic anticoagulation. The uninterrupted strategy also enables the avoidance of INR fluctuations, which are common and long lasting after VKA interruption (and which increase the risk of both thromboembolism and bleeding as well

Table 4.1 Peri-procedural anticoagulation regimens in OAC patients	
Uninterrupted VKA (pre-procedure INR 2.0–2.5)	Recommended*
VKA interruption (pre-procedure INR <1.8) with/without§ IV UFH/SC LMWH (enoxaparin) bridging	Accepted
NOAC interruption without IV UFH/SC LMWH (enoxaparin) bridging^	Recommended
Uninterrupted NOAC with PCI performed at NOAC trough concentration levels#	Accepted
Uninterrupted NOAC	Not recommended**

INR = International Normalized Ratio; IV = intravenous; LMWH = low-molecular-weight heparin; NOAC = newer, non-vitamin K antagonist, direct oral anticoagulant; OAC = oral anticoagulation; PCI = percutaneous coronary intervention; SC = subcutaneous; UFH = unfractionated heparin; VKA = vitamin K antagonist

* With possible exception of procedures at high risk of coronary perforation (recanalization of chronic total occlusion).

§ Depending on the thromboembolic risk of the condition for which OAC is indicated.

^ Provided that NOAC interruption is performed close to PCI (one to two days with normal renal function, three to four days with impaired renal function).

Approximately 12 and 24 h after the last intake of dabigatran or apixaban, and rivaroxaban, respectively.

** Accepted in emergency procedures (primary PCI for ST-elevation myocardial infarction).

Table 4.2 Intra-procedural IV additional anticoagulation in patients on uninterrupted therapeutic OAC

	Stable IHD and/or non-high-risk lesion		ACS and/or high-risk lesion#	
	VKA	NOAC&	VKA	NOAC
UFH/LMWH	Not recommended	Recommended*	Recommended*	Recommended*
Bivalirudin	Not recommended	Not recommended	May be considered§	May be considered§

ACS = acute coronary syndrome; IHD = ischaemic heart disease; IV = intravenous; LMWH = low-molecular-weight heparin; NOAC = newer, non-vitamin K antagonist, direct oral anticoagulant; OAC = oral anticoagulation; UFH = unfractionated heparin; VKA = vitamin K antagonist

Ulceration, superimposed thrombus, ostial, bifurcation, degenerated saphenous vein grafts.

* At reduced dose (UFH 30–50 U/kg, enoxaparin 0.3 mg/kg).

§ In ACS patients.

& When not timely interrupted.

as necessitating prolonged bridging therapy) and the transient prothrombotic state due to the suppression of proteins C and S occurring upon VKA re-initiation. In addition, because of the rapid reversal of anticoagulation obtained with the administration of prothrombin complex concentrates and/or vitamin K, the fear of 'unopposed' bleeding during therapeutic OAC with VKA should not be overemphasized. Of note, reversal of the anticoagulant effect of enoxaparin and fondaparinux, which are the recommended anticoagulants in acute coronary syndromes (ACS), may also be cumbersome, as protamine sulphate (the established antidote to UFH) has little or no effect, respectively, in neutralizing the above agents. To increase the safety of PCI during therapeutic OAC with VKA, the pre-procedural INR should aim at the lower end of the therapeutic range (2.0–2.5). Additional IV UFH or enoxaparin, which is required upon the start of PCI in the ordinary patient, should only be given, and at a reduced dose (UFH, 30–50 U/kg; enoxaparin, 0.3 mg/kg), to those patients on therapeutic OAC with VKA undergoing PCI of high-risk lesions and/or in the context of ACS (where the thrombotic stimulus is stronger and/or the thrombus burden larger). As they appear to provide no additional benefit, while possibly increasing bleeding complications, additional IV UFH or enoxaparin should not be given to elective patients with stable ischaemic heart disease (IHD) undergoing PCI of non-high-risk lesions.

Alternatively, OAC with VKA may be interrupted prior (approximately five days) to PCI and may or may not (depending on the thromboembolic risk of the condition requiring OAC) be bridged with IV UFH or SC enoxaparin. The interrupted strategy should aim at a pre-procedural INR <1.8, and standard-dose IV UFH or enoxaparin should be given upon the start of PCI. Because of the need for temporary heparin bridging during VKA interruption, such a strategy is associated with prolonged hospital stay and, hence, increased costs; and it also contributes to the longer waiting times for PCI which have been reported for ACS patients receiving VKA.

In patients on OAC with NOAC, interruption should generally be preferred over continuation. Dabigatran appears to provide insufficient anticoagulation during PCI in stable IHD, and the absence of easy and reliable quantitative laboratory monitoring, as well as the lack of antidote, make the peri-procedural management of NOAC more problematic. On the other hand, the favourable pharmacokinetics of NOAC, allowing for rapid offset and onset of the effect, make the discontinuation strategy convenient. The time of NOAC discontinuation should be guided by the half-life of each drug, allowing for interruption close to the procedure (one to two days with normal renal function, three to four days with impaired renal function) without IV UFH or SC enoxaparin bridging. When OAC interruption is performed within 24–48 h of the surgical or invasive procedure, the incidence of peri-procedural major bleeding appears lower with NOAC compared to VKA, in the absence of differences in peri-procedural thromboembolism. The standard dose of UFH (70–100 U/kg) or enoxaparin (0.5–0.75 mg/kg) should be given upon the start of PCI when NOAC have been discontinued in a timely manner. Early (same day of intervention) restarting of NOAC after PCI should then be performed, again without UFH or enoxaparin bridging because of the rapid (two to four hours) onset of action. Restarting however, should be performed ≥4 h after the last dose of UFH and ≥8 h after the last dose of enoxaparin, as by that time the anticoagulant effect of these drugs would be disappearing.

Alternatively, in patients on OAC with NOAC, consideration should be given to perform PCI at the trough concentration levels (about 12 and 24 h from the last intake of dabigatran or apixaban, and rivaroxaban, respectively) without drug interruption. Although specific data are lacking, it is reasonable in these cases to give reduced-dose IV UFH (30–50 U/kg) or enoxaparin (0.3 mg/kg) at the beginning of PCI.

Performance of PCI during ongoing NOAC is both unavoidable and accepted in the emergency setting of primary PCI for ST-elevation myocardial infarction (STEMI). Regardless of the time elapsed from the last intake of NOAC, reduced-dose of IV UFH (30–50 U/kg) or enoxaparin (0.3 mg/kg) should be given upon the start of PCI.

IV administration of the direct thrombin inhibitor bivalirudin is increasingly used in PCI for ACS, as, compared to the standard treatment of combined IV UFH and glycoprotein IIb/IIIa inhibitors (GPI), it is associated with similar MACE and stroke rate but lower bleeding. Because of that, bivalirudin may be considered as IV anticoagulant in patients on ongoing therapeutic OAC (with either VKA or NOAC) undergoing PCI for ACS, although specific data on the efficacy and safety of this strategy are currently lacking.

4.1.2 Antiplatelet therapy (Table 4.3)

Similarly to ordinary patients and those patients on OAC undergoing PCI, antiplatelet therapy is warranted to prevent peri-procedural ischaemic events and stent thrombosis. In general, DAPT with aspirin and a $P2Y_{12}$-receptor inhibitor is recommended.

Table 4.3 Antiplatelet drugs for PCI in OAC patients		
Aspirin		Recommended*
$P2Y_{12}$-receptor inhibitors	Clopidogrel	Recommended**
	Prasugrel^	Not recommended
	Ticagrelor^	Not recommended
GPI	Abciximab, eptifibatide, tirofiban	Not recommended#

ACS = acute coronary syndrome; GPI = glycoprotein IIb/IIIa inhibitors; OAC = oral anticoagulation; PCI = percutaneous coronary intervention

* Loading dose 150–325 mg orally (PO) ≥2 h (ideally ≥24 h) before or 80–150 mg IV upon start + maintenance dose 75–100 mg/day.

** Loading dose 300 mg PO (or alternatively 600 mg, depending on the time of scheduled PCI and/or risk of bleeding of patient) + maintenance dose 75 mg/day.

May be considered (in patients on OAC with VKA) only when International Normalized Ratio (INR) ≤2.0.

^ ACS patients only.

Aspirin should be given as with the ordinary patient. In contrast, consideration should be given as to whether to administer a 300 or 600 mg loading dose of clopidogrel. Whereas no specific data comparing the safety and efficacy of the two doses are available for VKA patients, it is known that the 600 mg dose is associated with a more rapid and intense platelet inhibition. The 300 or 600 mg loading dose should then be chosen based on the time scheduled for PCI and/or the bleeding risk of the patient. Because the risk of bleeding in VKA patients is increased due to the combination of antithrombotic therapies, the lower 300 mg loading dose should generally be preferred.

The combination of aspirin with newer $P2Y_{12}$-receptor inhibitors (prasugrel, ticagrelor), which provide a more potent and predictable antiplatelet effect than clopidogrel at the cost, however, of increased major bleeding, should be avoided in patients on OAC with VKA. For the above reason as well as the lack of data, prasugrel and ticagrelor should not be combined with NOAC either.

GPI should generally not be used in patients on OAC with VKA, owing to the reported more than five-fold increase in the risk of early major bleeding, with up to 20% of patients experiencing a major bleed when the femoral access is used. Because of that, these agents should be avoided in VKA patients and only considered when the INR ≤2.0. Owing to the neutral effect on the incidence of major bleeding (and MACE) of the intracoronary administration of abciximab as bolus only rather than the conventional IV bolus plus infusion, the intracoronary route is of uncertain value in reducing the risk of bleeding in OAC patients and therefore is not routinely recommended. No data are available regarding the adjunct of GPI in patients on ongoing NOAC, and therefore such a combination should generally be avoided.

4.1.3 Technique

Because of both the enormous reduction of in-hospital bleeding and the vascular access-site complications observed in large datasets of ordinary patients, as well as in small groups of patients on VKA, when PCI is performed via the *radial route*, this vascular access should be preferred in patients on therapeutic OAC, provided that adequate expertise is available. Indeed, the femoral route is a major independent predictor of access-site complications, with up to a ten-fold increase in VKA patients undergoing PCI. Whenever the radial approach is not feasible, ongoing therapeutic OAC should not exclude the femoral approach, provided that the puncture is carefully carried out according to the proper technique (common femoral artery, anterior artery wall only), and possibly under ultrasound guidance.

No data are currently available on the efficacy and safety of *vascular closure devices (VCD)* for femoral haemostasis in patients on therapeutic OAC undergoing PCI. Even though manual compression has been shown to be feasible and safe in VKA patients undergoing coronary angiography, the use of VCD is systematically advised following PCI. Allowing earlier haemostasis and ambulation, and hence earlier hospital discharge, VCD have also been shown to be effective in reducing access-site bleeding complications in ordinary patients at increased risk of peri-procedural bleeding and/or submitted to aggressive antithrombotic therapy (with whom OAC patients may be assimilated).

Among adjunctive therapeutic devices, *aspiration thrombectomy* should be considered in patients on OAC undergoing primary PCI for STEMI. Even though data on OAC patients are lacking, thrombus removal by manual aspiration in a setting where the thrombus burden is generally large and aggressive antithrombotic therapy with additional anticoagulants and antiplatelet agents (namely GPI) is hindered by the increased risk of bleeding may help in reducing distal embolization and no-reflow.

4.1.4 Stents (Table 4.4)

Because of the indication for a shorter duration of DAPT (one vs 6–12 months) and therefore the decreased risk of bleeding associated with a shorter exposure to combination therapy of OAC and antiplatelets, in OAC patients undergoing PCI the implantation of bare-metal stents (BMS) should be generally preferred over that of drug-eluting stents (DES). Yet, DES may be considered for and strictly limited to those clinical (diabetes, chronic kidney disease) and/or anatomical (long lesions, small vessels, chronic total occlusion, in-stent restenosis) conditions where the risk of restenosis is higher and a higher benefit compared to BMS is expected. When DES are chosen, new-generation everolimus- or zotarolimus-DES should be preferred because of the lower risk of stent thrombosis and the associated possibility to shorten (≤3-6 months) DAPT. Also, implantation of new-generation polymer-reabsorbable or polymer–free DES, as well as of bioresorbable vascular scaffolds (BVS), which undergo degradation over time, may be considered to keep the duration of DAPT <12 months. Implantation of new-generation DES, however, should not necessarily imply a shorter prescription of DAPT but should instead allow safe earlier DAPT interruption in the event that clinically significant bleeding occurs.

Whereas specific data on the so-called 'bio-active' stents (BAS), including diamond-like carbon- and titanium nitric oxide-coated stents in OAC patients are lacking, consideration may be given to these stents, owing to their higher biocompatibility, which in turn may be associated with a lower risk of stent thrombosis (as well as of restenosis), likely allowing for a duration of DAPT as short as a few (two to four) weeks. Similarly, paclitaxel-coated drug-eluting balloons (DEB), for which DAPT duration as short as one month appears sufficient, may be considered in these patients.

Table 4.4 Type of stent/scaffold for PCI in OAC patients			
BMS			Recommended*
DES	Early-generation	Sirolimus-, paclitaxel-eluting	Not recommended
	New-generation	Everolimus-, zotarolimus-eluting (durable polymer)	Accepted#
		Biolimus A9™-eluting (bioabsorbable polymer)	Accepted
		Amphilimus™-eluting (polymer-free)	Accepted
BAS		Diamond-like carbon-, titanium nitric oxide-coated	Accepted
		Endothelial progenitor cells-capturing	Not recommended
BVS		Non-drug-eluting	Accepted
		Everolimus-, myolimus-, sirolimus-eluting	Accepted

BAS = bio-active stents; BMS = bare-metal stents; BVS = bioresorbable vascular scaffolds; DES = drug-eluting stents; OAC = oral anticoagulation; PCI = percutaneous coronary intervention

* To be generally preferred.

\# To be considered in clinical (diabetes, chronic kidney disease) and/or anatomical (long lesions, small vessels, chronic total occlusion, in-stent restenosis) conditions at higher risk of restenosis.

No data are currently available regarding the choice of stent in patients on NOAC, and therefore the same recommendations for patients on VKA should be followed.

In Figure 4.1, a comprehensive peri-procedural strategy to optimize the efficacy-to-safety balance of PCI in OAC patients is outlined.

4.1.5 Adverse events (Table 4.5)

The absolute peri-procedural incidence of thromboembolism, stent thrombosis, MACE, and bleeding in OAC patients undergoing PCI is difficult to estimate because of the different definitions used (particularly regarding bleeding) and the many variables involved. Also, available data derive from heterogeneous populations where OAC has often been interrupted prior to PCI, which was therefore carried out under ordinary conditions (DAPT, and anticoagulation with UFH/enoxaparin or bivalirudin). Procedural variables, including vascular access site, management of anticoagulation, and use of GPI, may also substantially impact on the occurrence of early bleeding complications. Whereas it is uncertain whether the peri-procedural incidence of thromboembolism, stent thrombosis, and MACE is higher in OAC compared to ordinary patients, access-site complications (when the femoral approach is used) and bleeding tend to be more frequent.

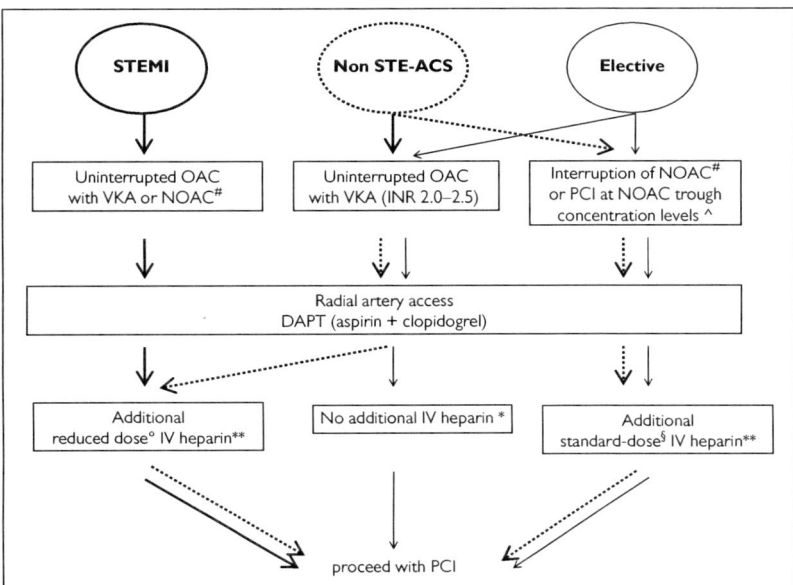

Figure 4.1 General procedural algorithm to optimize the efficacy-to-safety balance of PCI in patients on OAC (with VKA or NOAC).

ACS = acute coronary syndrome; non-STE-ACS = non-ST-elevation acute coronary syndrome; DAPT = dual antiplatelet therapy; STEMI = STE myocardial infarction; ^ about 12 and 24 h from the last intake of dabigatran or apixaban, and rivaroxaban, respectively; # thrombin inhibitor dabigatran, factor Xa inhibitors rivaroxaban, and apixaban; * except for high-risk lesions, where reduced-dose UFH/enoxaparin should be given; ° UFH, 30–50 U/kg or enoxaparin, 0.3 mg/kg; § UFH, 70–100 U/kg or enoxaparin, 0.5–0.75 mg/kg; ** bivalirudin may be considered (ACS).

Table 4.5 Peri-procedural incidence of adverse events in OAC patients undergoing PCI

Adverse event		(%)
MACE	death	2.0
	myocardial infarction	1.5
	emergency bypass surgery	1.5
Stroke		0.5
Stent thrombosis		0.7
Clinically significant bleeding^		2.0–3.0
Blood transfusions		1.5
Vascular complications (femoral approach)		8.0

OAC = oral anticoagulation; MACE = major adverse cardiac events; PCI = percutaneous coronary intervention
^ Prompting evaluation and/or treatment, or fatal.

Limited data are available on the peri-procedural event rate of patients on NOAC undergoing PCI. The incidence of bleeding, however, appears lower with NOAC compared to VKA when drug discontinuation has been carried out in the proximity (24–48 h) of the procedure.

4.2 Post-procedural issues and long-term management

The post-procedural management of OAC patients undergoing PCI should aim at limiting the risks of a) thromboembolism (stroke or systemic embolism, pulmonary embolism) associated with the clinical condition requiring OAC, b) stent thrombosis inherent to the implantation of a coronary stent, and c) MACE, which characterize the natural history of IHD, while d) minimizing at the same time the risk of bleeding. The antithrombotic therapy should be selected based on the individual risk of thromboembolism and carefully managed throughout based on the individual risk of bleeding. Additional management and/or pharmacological measures might be adopted to further optimize the balance between efficacy and safety of the antithrombotic therapy.

4.2.1 Antithrombotic therapy

The selection of the antithrombotic regimen should start from the stratification of the risk of thromboembolism associated with the clinical condition requiring OAC (Table 4.6).

In patients at moderate-to-high (2–10% and above per year) risk of thromboembolism, OAC (with VKA) is warranted after PCI owing to the established inferiority of DAPT (which is recommended after PCI) in preventing thromboembolism. In turn, OAC (with VKA) is inferior to DAPT in preventing stent thrombosis and MACE following PCI. Thus, a combined antithrombotic therapy with OAC (with VKA) and DAPT is required. Triple therapy (TT) with VKA, aspirin, and clopidogrel has been consistently shown to provide superior coverage to both DAPT and the combination of VKA with single antiplatelet therapy (SAPT; using either aspirin or clopidogrel) against thromboembolism, stent thrombosis, and MACE. According to initial data, the combination of VKA and SAPT with clopidogrel may have both superior safety (occurrence of total

Table 4.6 Absolute risk of thromboembolism of clinical indications for OAC

Risk	Incidence/year (%)	OAC indication
High	4–10 and above	AF (CHA$_2$DS$_2$-VASc score ≥4) Previous cardiogenic stroke/systemic embolism Mechanical heart valve Biological mitral or tricuspid valve (<3 months from implantation) Intracardiac thrombus Recent (<3–6 months) VTE Recurrent VTE Thrombophilia
Moderate	2–3	AF (CHA$_2$DS$_2$-VASc score 2–3)
		Previous (6–12 months) VTE*
Low	<2	AF (CHA$_2$DS$_2$-VASc score 1)
		Previous (>12 months) VTE*

AF = atrial fibrillation; CHA$_2$DS$_2$-VASc = **C**ongestive heart failure, **H**ypertension, **A**ge ≥75 years, **D**iabetes, **S**troke, associated **V**ascular disease, **A**ge 65–74 years, **S**ex category; OAC = oral anticoagulation; VTE = venous thromboembolism

* In the absence of risk factors for recurrence (unprovoked, recurrent episodes, thrombophilia, cancer).

bleeding) and efficacy (combined occurrence of stroke, MACE, and stent thrombosis) compared to TT. Because such data are not conclusive regarding the real efficacy, especially against stent thrombosis, of the combination of VKA and clopidogrel, this regimen is currently not recommended. In contrast, the combination of VKA and aspirin has long been demonstrated to be suboptimal in preventing stent thrombosis and MACE after PCI and is therefore contraindicated. Given the paucity of data, the combination of VKA and newer P2Y$_{12}$-receptor inhibitors (prasugrel, ticagrelor), either with or without aspirin, is not recommended as well. Limited evidence suggests that post-discharge TT of VKA, aspirin, and prasugrel is associated with a substantial (fourfold) increase in overall bleeding compared with the conventional TT of VKA, aspirin, and clopidogrel. Thus, whenever an indication for OAC arises in patients on DAPT with aspirin and newer P2Y$_{12}$-receptor inhibitors (prasugrel, ticagrelor), these latter should be substituted by clopidogrel for as long as TT is required.

In patients at low (about 1% per year) risk of thromboembolism, a short (between one and three to six months, depending on whether a BMS or DES has been implanted, and/or PCI has been performed in stable IHD or ACS) course of DAPT is generally preferable over TT. In selected patients at very low bleeding risk, however, a similarly short course of TT may be considered instead.

TT should always be considered to carry an increased risk of overall bleeding and should therefore be reserved for those patients for whom the expected net clinical benefit is favourable. Thus, TT should not be denied because of an increased risk of bleeding to patients at a moderate-to-high risk of thromboembolisms, as in these patients the overall benefit of TT appears not to be outweighed by a high bleeding risk. In contrast, in patients at low thromboembolic risk, the decision to give TT over DAPT should be guided by the individual risk of bleeding, as the higher efficacy of TT in reducing an already low risk of thromboembolism might be outweighed by an increase in the risk of bleeding. In selected patients at high thromboembolic risk in whom the bleeding risk is deemed too high for even a short (two to four weeks) course of TT, such a regimen is not suitable, and alternative management strategies (balloon angioplasty without stent implantation, bypass surgery, medical therapy) should be considered.

Because of the considerations above, assessment of bleeding risk, either empirical or assisted by stratification schemas, should be carried out together with the assessment of thromboembolic risk at the time of selecting the antithrombotic therapy. Such initial bleeding-risk stratification, together with its periodical reassessment, will also help to guide the subsequent management of antithrombotic therapy and establish the level of care throughout treatment. Among the several available risk-of-bleeding stratification schemas, the HAS-BLED (**H**ypertension, **A**bnormal liver or kidney function, prior **S**troke, **B**leeding history or predisposition, **L**abile INR, **E**lderly, concomitant **D**rugs) score, appears the most practical and the best predictor. Although having been initially developed and validated in patients with AF and exhibiting only an absolute modest predictive ability, the HAS-BLED score has been shown to be applicable also to patients receiving TT after an ACS.

In Figure 4.2, a comprehensive strategy for the selection of antithrombotic therapy is outlined.

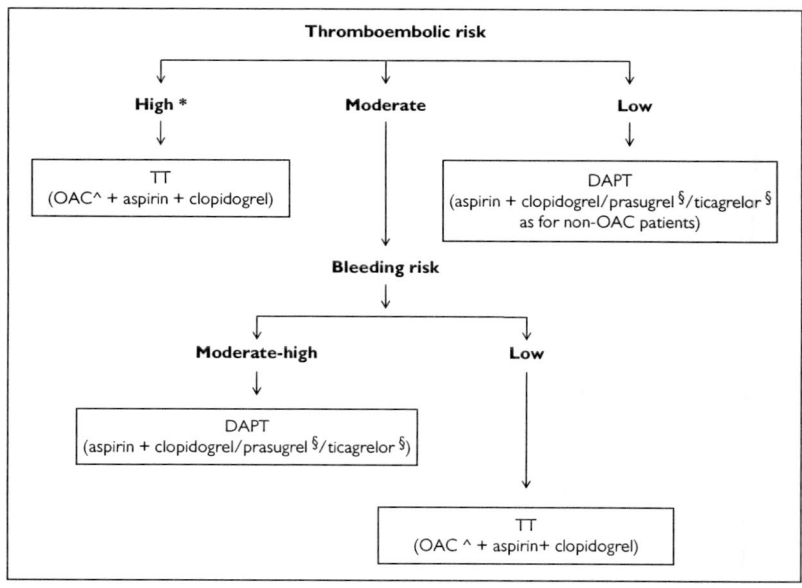

Figure 4.2 Choice of post-discharge antithrombotic regimen.

ACS = acute coronary syndrome; DAPT = dual antiplatelet therapy; OAC = oral anticoagulation; TT = triple therapy.

* Whenever the bleeding risk is considered too high even for a short (two to four weeks) course of triple therapy, alternative strategies, such as balloon angioplasty without stent implantation, or bypass surgery, or medical treatment, rather than alternative antithrombotic regimens, should be considered; ^with either VKA or NOAC; §ACS only.

Little data are currently available on the combination of NOAC, aspirin, and clopidogrel. Because of that, TT of NOAC, aspirin, and clopidogrel is not routinely recommended, and VKA should generally be preferred over NOAC when the indication for OAC arises in a patient already on DAPT. In patients who are on NOAC at the time of PCI, it is reasonable to continue NOAC rather than substitute them with VKA, owing to the initial reports of comparable safety of the combination of VKA or NOAC (dabigatran) with DAPT and the known increase in the risk of bleeding during switching between antithrombotic agents. The lower dose of the NOAC (dabigatran, 110 mg twice daily; rivaroxaban, 15 mg once daily; apixaban, 2.5 mg twice daily) should preferably be used together with DAPT for as long as TT is required.

Similar to VKA, the combination of NOAC with newer $P2Y_{12}$-receptor inhibitors (prasugrel, ticagrelor), with or without aspirin, should be avoided, owing both to the lack of data and the reported increase of bleeding with VKA, aspirin, and prasugrel.

An overview of the various antithrombotic regimens is reported in Table 4.7.

4.2.2 Management of antithrombotic therapy

Once the antithrombotic therapy (namely TT) has been selected after PCI, maximal care should be given to ensure the optimal balance between prevention of thromboembolism, stent thrombosis, and MACE, while avoiding bleeding. Avoidance of bleeding is of paramount importance, not only because when major it may be life-threatening or even fatal (intracranial, causing shock) but also because even when minor it may induce caregivers to withdraw the antithrombotic agents, leaving therefore the patient exposed to potentially catastrophic consequences (stroke, pulmonary embolism, stent thrombosis). Apart from the established clinical factors for bleeding (advanced age, previous stroke/bleeding, hypertension, anaemia, diabetes, abnormal renal/liver function), which are incorporated in most of the bleeding risk stratification schemas, the

Table 4.7 Antithrombotic regimens for OAC patients at moderate-to-high TE risk undergoing PCI		
TT	VKA + aspirin + clopidogrel	Recommended
	VKA/NOAC + aspirin + prasugrel/ticagrelor	Not recommended
	NOAC + aspirin + clopidogrel	Accepted*
OAC + SAPT	VKA/NOAC + aspirin	Contraindicated
	VKA + clopidogrel	Not recommended
	NOAC + clopidogrel	Not recommended
	VKA/NOAC + prasugrel/ticagrelor	Not recommended
DAPT	aspirin + clopidogrel	Accepted⁸
	aspirin + prasugrel/ticagrelor	Accepted⁸^

ACS = acute coronary syndrome; DAPT = dual antiplatelet therapy; NOAC = newer, non-vitamin K antagonist, direct oral anticoagulant; OAC = oral anticoagulation; PCI = percutaneous coronary intervention; SAPT = single antiplatelet therapy; TE = thromboembolic; TT = triple therapy; VKA = vitamin K antagonist

* In patients already on a NOAC, and provided that the lower dose (dabigatran, 110 mg twice daily; rivaroxaban, 15 mg once daily; apixaban, 2.5 mg twice daily) is given for the duration of TT.

⁸ When TE risk is moderate (atrial fibrillation with CHA_2DS_2-VASc score 1-2, VTE within 6–12 months without risk factors for recurrence) and bleeding risk is increased.

^ ACS only.

risk of bleeding during antithrombotic therapy is influenced by several other variables, including the duration and intensity of the antithrombotic therapy.

The exposure to TT may impact on the incidence of bleeding, with a reported major bleeding rate of about 3, 6, and 8% at one, six, and 12 months, respectively. Thus, TT should be given for as short a period of time as possible, particularly in patients at increased risk of bleeding. Such a recommendation is even more stringent when TT is carried out with NOAC, aspirin, and clopidogrel because of the still largely unknown benefit-to-risk balance of such a combination.

The intensity of TT may also impact on the incidence of bleeding, and therefore the lowest possible dose of antithrombotic drugs should be used. Aspirin should be given at a dose ≤100 mg/day, and clopidogrel, at the dose of 75 mg/day. The INR, when OAC is carried out with VKA, should be maintained at the lower end of the therapeutic range (2.0–2.5). When OAC is carried out with NOAC, the lower dose (dabigatran, 110 mg twice daily; rivaroxaban, 15 mg once daily; apixaban, 2.5 mg twice daily) should be used.

As an additional measure aiming to increase the safety of TT combining DAPT with VKA or NOAC, close monitoring of INR (every two weeks) or renal function, complete blood count, and haemoglobin (every four weeks) respectively should be arranged.

During TT, most bleeding is gastrointestinal (GI); therefore, gastric protection should be routinely administered. Because proton-pump inhibitors (PPI) are more effective than H_2–receptor inhibitors in reducing the risk of upper GI bleeding, they should generally be preferred. PPI (pantoprazole) not interfering with the cytochrome P450 (CYP) 2C19, which is key in converting the prodrug clopidogrel into its active metabolite, should preferably be selected, as those (omeprazole, esomeprazole) interfering with CYP2C19 may reduce the efficacy of clopidogrel and consequently increase the risk of stent thrombosis and MACE. Of note, the H_2-inhibitor cimetidine (but not ranitidine) also interferes with CYP2C19 and should therefore be avoided.

Owing to the increased risk of bleeding, concomitant use of non-steroidal anti-inflammatory drugs should be avoided throughout TT.

An overview of the strategies to reduce the risk of bleeding during TT is reported in Table 4.8.

Following the initial between one to three-six months course of TT with VKA, aspirin, and clopidogrel (depending on whether a BMS or DES has been implanted and/or PCI has been performed in stable IHD or ACS), one antiplatelet drug (either aspirin or clopidogrel) may be discontinued (because of the decreased risk of stent thrombosis) and a combination of VKA and SAPT administered for up to 12 months (after which the risk of MACE is also substantially decreased). Whereas either aspirin or clopidogrel may be maintained together with VKA, the combination of VKA and aspirin is generally preferable owing to an apparently lower risk of bleeding. Routine gastric protection, as well as a low dose of the antiplatelet agent, is warranted also in this phase, whereas targeting the INR to the lower end of therapeutic range (2.0–2.5) vs standard therapeutic range (2.0–3.0) should be individualized.

In patients at low thromboembolic risk in whom DAPT has been chosen for the initial phase of between one and three to six months (depending on whether a BMS or DES has been implanted and/or PCI has been performed in stable IHD or ACS), VKA should be restarted after one antiplatelet agent (either aspirin or clopidogrel) has been withdrawn, and the subsequent management should be carried out as above.

No detailed data are available regarding the medium- to long-term management of PCI patients receiving TT with NOAC, aspirin, and clopidogrel. Because of that and

Table 4.8 Strategies to reduce the risk of bleeding with TT (and antithrombotic therapies in general)

Short duration	1-month:	With BMS in stable IHD*
	3-month:	With DES° in stable IHD
		With BMS/DES° in ACS^
Low treatment intensity	Low-dose aspirin:	≤100 mg/day
	Low-dose clopidogrel:	75 mg/day
	Lower therapeutic end INR (with VKA):	2.0–2.5
	Lower dose of NOAC:	Dabigatran, 110 mg twice daily
		Rivaroxaban, 15 mg once daily
		Apixaban, 2.5 mg twice daily
Frequent monitoring	INR (with VKA):	Every 2 weeks
	Clinical and/or laboratory& (with NOAC):	Every 4 weeks
Gastric protection	Proton-pump inhibitors:	Pantoprazole 20–40 mg/day
	H₂-inhibitors:	Ranitidine 300-600 mg/day
Avoidance of NSAID	—	—

ACS = acute coronary syndrome; BMS = bare-metal stents; DES = drug-eluting stents; IHD = ischaemic heart disease; INR = International Normalized Ratio; NOAC = newer, non-vitamin K antagonist, direct oral anticoagulant; NSAID = non-steroidal anti-inflammatory drugs; TT = triple therapy; VKA = vitamin K antagonist

* Two weeks only may be considered in occasional patients at very high bleeding risk.

° New-generation (everolimus- or zotarolimus-eluting, polymer-bioabsorbable or polymer-free).

^ Six to 12 months may be considered in patients at very low risk of bleeding.

& Renal function, blood cell count, and haemoglobin.

the reported comparable safety of the combination of either NOAC (dabigatran) or VKA and SAPT (mostly aspirin), with no interaction with the efficacy observed without concomitant antiplatelet therapy, the same strategy as above is advised. Depending on the estimated individual risk of bleeding, the dose of the NOAC, which had been reduced at the start of TT and maintained at the reduced level throughout TT, may be returned to the standard dose (dabigatran, 150 mg twice daily; rivaroxaban, 20 mg once daily; apixaban, 5 mg twice daily), unless a previous indication for the reduced dose (increased risk of bleeding, renal impairment) is present.

After 12 months of PCI, ongoing SAPT should be stopped and OAC alone with either VKA or NOAC continued indefinitely at the individual appropriate INR range or dose.

Given the present lack of data, an extended duration of >12 months of combined OAC and SAPT with either aspirin or clopidogrel may only be considered when the risk of potentially catastrophic consequences in the event of stent thrombosis is high (left main, last remaining vessel) and the risk of bleeding is low.

The recommendations for antithrombotic therapy following PCI are summarized in Table 4.9.

In Figure 4.3, an algorithm summarizing the general management of patients on OAC (with either VKA or NOAC) undergoing PCI in the context of an ACS is outlined.

Table 4.9 Recommendations for the various antithrombotic strategies following PCI

	Time frame	Setting
TT (OAC[&], aspirin and clopidogrel)	1 month	BMS in stable IHD[*]
	3–6 months	DES[°] in stable IHD
		BMS/DES[°] in ACS[^]
OAC[&] + aspirin[§]	after 1 to 3–6 months and up to 12 months	All cases
OAC[&] alone[#]	after 12 months and indefinitely	All cases

ACS = acute coronary syndrome; BMS = bare-metal stents; DES = drug-eluting stents; IHD = ischaemic heart disease; NOAC = newer, non-vitamin K antagonist, direct oral anticoagulant; OAC = oral anticoagulation; PCI = percutaneous coronary intervention; VKA = vitamin K antagonist

[&] With VKA or NOAC (if they were previously ongoing).

[§] Clopidogrel instead of aspirin acceptable.

[*] Two weeks only may be considered in occasional patients at very high bleeding risk.

[°] New-generation everolimus- or zotarolimus-eluting, polymer-bioabsorbable, or polymer-free.

[^] Six to 12 months may be considered in patients at very low risk of bleeding.

[#] Regular intensity to be reinstituted: INR 2.0–3.0 for most patients on VKA or dabigatran, 150 mg twice daily, rivaroxaban, 15 mg once daily, apixaban, 5 mg twice daily (unless indication for reduced intensity was previously present).

4.2.3 Adverse events

An accurate estimation of the post-discharge rate of thromboembolism, stent thrombosis, and MACE in OAC patients undergoing PCI and treated with the recommended antithrombotic regimen (namely TT) is difficult, as different definitions of the adverse events, and particularly of bleeding, have been used. Furthermore, most data derive from retrospective, small datasets, where the antithrombotic therapy actually ongoing at the time of an adverse (thromboembolic or bleeding) event and the corresponding INR value (in case of VKA treatment) are seldom reported. Also, the incidence of adverse events, and particularly bleeding, during follow up has only rarely been reported separately from the in-hospital rate (which is more affected by procedural variables than by ongoing antithrombotic treatment), therefore making difficult a reliable estimation of the absolute, as well as relative, incidence of adverse events.

Based on the comparable, or even lower, incidence of thromboembolism and bleeding with NOAC compared with VKA in AF and venous thromboembolism, as well as the comparable incidence of bleeding with NOAC (dabigatran) and VKA when combined with antiplatelets, with no interaction with the incidence of thromboembolism observed without concomitant antiplatelet therapy, the medium- to long-term efficacy and safety of TT with either VKA or NOAC, aspirin, and clopidogrel should be considered substantially similar.

An estimation of the absolute 12-month occurrence of adverse events in PCI patients receiving TT is reported in Table 4.10.

Whereas the substantial rate of MACE generally reported in OAC patients undergoing PCI may be related to the established greater frailty of OAC patients, the relevant incidence of bleeding is likely due to the aggressive antithrombotic therapy (namely TT). Of note, a larger proportion of bleeding events is accounted for by non-major bleeding, whereas some uncertainty exists over whether major bleeding is also substantially increased. Nonetheless, non-major bleeding must be regarded to be of clinical importance, as it may induce caregivers to withdraw the antithrombotic agents, therefore increasing the risk of thromboembolism, stent thrombosis, and MACE. Accurate

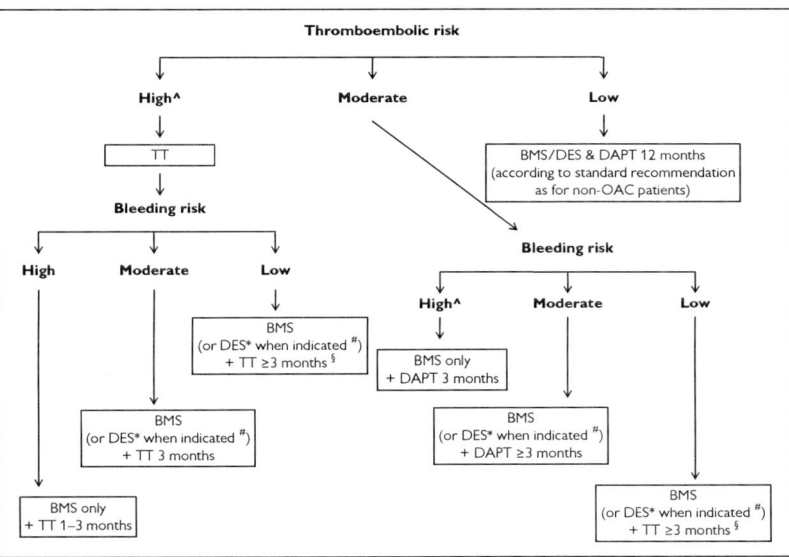

Figure 4.3 Algorithm for the management of patients on OAC undergoing PCI in the context of an ACS.

BMS = bare-metal stents; DAPT = dual antiplatelet therapy; DES = drug-eluting stents; OAC = oral anticoagulation; TT = triple therapy; ^ Whenever the bleeding risk is considered too high for a three-month course of triple therapy, alternative strategies, such as balloon angioplasty without stent implantation, bypass surgery, or medical treatment, rather than alternative antithrombotic regimens, should be considered; * new-generation (everolimus- or zotarolimus-eluting, polymer-bioabsorbable or polymer-free) recommended; # in clinical (diabetes, chronic kidney disease) and/or anatomical (long lesions, small vessels, chronic total occlusion, in-stent restenosis) at increased risk of restenosis; § up to 6–12 months.

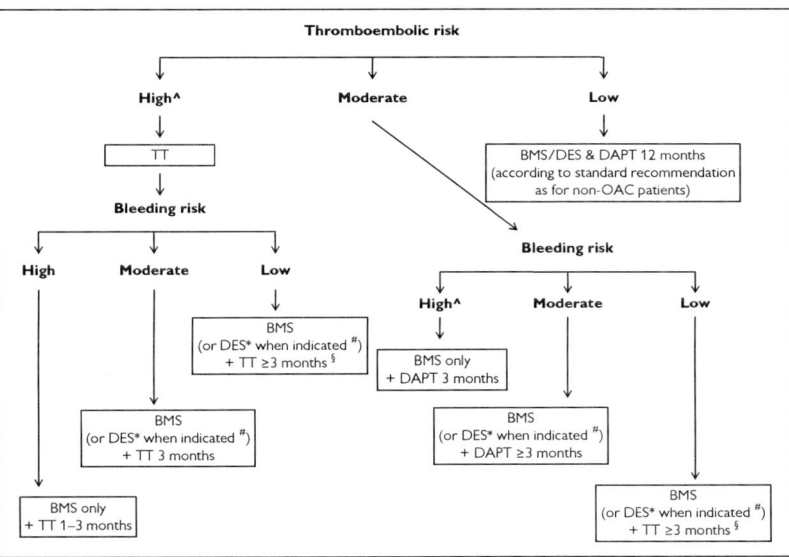

Table 4.10 Twelve-month incidence of adverse events in OAC patients undergoing PCI and receiving TT

Adverse event		(%)
MACE:	death	5
	myocardial infarction	3
	TVR/TLR	4
Stroke		<1
Stent thrombosis		<1
MACE + stroke + stent thrombosis		9
Major bleeding		6
Non-major bleeding		9
All bleeding		15

MACE = major adverse cardiac events; OAC = oral anticoagulation; PCI = percutaneous coronary intervention; TLR = target lesion revascularization; TT = triple therapy; TVR = target vessel revascularization assessment of both thromboembolic and bleeding risk, judicious selection of the most appropriate antithrombotic regimen, and careful subsequent management are warranted to limit the occurrence of even minor bleeding.

4.3 Management of bleeding (Table 4.11)

Owing to the concomitant risk of thromboembolism, stent thrombosis, and MACE, the management of bleeding in OAC patients undergoing PCI is complex. Variables including time elapsed from PCI (less than vs more than one to three months), type of stent implanted (BMS vs DES vs other), severity (major vs non-major) and location (intracranial vs internal vs external) of bleeding, and ongoing antithrombotic therapy at the event (TT vs OAC and SAPT vs OAC only), as well as type of ongoing OAC (VKA vs NOAC), influence the modalities of treatment. Thus, measures ranging from watchful waiting to interruption of all antithrombotic agents may be adopted.

Whenever bleeding is deemed clinically relevant, VKA should immediately be interrupted and subsequently managed as in ordinary VKA patients. Throughout the period most vulnerable to stent thrombosis (one month with BMS, three to six months with new-generation DES) during which TT is ongoing, great care should be given to not interrupting both aspirin and $P2Y_{12}$-receptor inhibitor at the same time because of the substantial risk of stent thrombosis. Either aspirin or clopidogrel should be discontinued in the event of clinically significant bleeding and promptly reinstituted as soon as adequate haemostasis has been obtained (and risk of recurrent bleeding is low). Following completion of the recommended course of TT (between one and three to six months or longer) and during combined therapy of VKA and SAPT (either aspirin or clopidogrel), withdrawal of both antithrombotic drugs appears feasible when necessary. Maintenance of the antiplatelet agent (generally aspirin), however, is always advisable to minimize the risk of stent thrombosis. The management of bleeding >12 months after PCI and during VKA therapy only should be carried out as in ordinary VKA patients.

Table 4.11 Strategies for the management of clinically significant bleeding following PCI			
	During TT	**During OAC* + SAPT**	**During OAC* only**
OAC* interruption	Recommended	Recommended	Recommended
OAC* reversal	To be considered ^	To be considered ^	To be considered ^
Withdrawal of both antiplatelets	Not recommended	—	—
Withdrawal of one antiplatelet	To be considered	To be considered	—
General measures to preserve circulation °	Recommended	Recommended	Recommended
Local (endoscopic/surgical) haemostasis#	Recommended	Recommended	Recommended

NOAC = newer, non-vitamin K antagonist, direct oral anticoagulant; OAC = oral anticoagulation; PCI = percutaneous coronary intervention; TT = triple therapy; VKA = vitamin K antagonist

* With either VKA or NOAC.

^ In life-threatening bleeding (intracranial).

° Plasma expanders, blood transfusions, inotropic support.

When feasible.

No data are currently available regarding the management of bleeding in patients on combined NOAC and antiplatelet agents. At present, the same strategy as above is recommended. Of note, a more rapid disappearance of the anticoagulant effect is to be expected after interruption of NOAC compared to VKA, owing to the more favourable pharmacokinetics.

Table 4.12 Overview of management preferences/recommendations

		VKA	NOAC
Peri-procedure			
OAC[&]		Continuation (INR ≥2.0)	Discontinuation [°] (w/o heparin bridging)
Additional heparin	Stable IHD/non high-risk lesion	No	Yes[§]
	ACS/high-risk lesion	Yes[*]	Yes[§]
GPI		No	No
Clopidogrel loading dose		300 mg	300 mg
Prasugrel, ticagrelor[**]		No	No
Bivalirudin[**]		No[$]	No[$]
Vascular access		Radial	Radial
Type of stent		BMS	BMS
Post-procedure			
Antithrombotic therapy		TT (VKA, aspirin, clopidogrel)	TT (NOAC, aspirin, clopidogrel)
Duration		1–3 months[#]	1–3 months[#]
Intensity of OAC		Lower INR (2.0–2.5)	Lower NOAC dose[^]
Monitoring		INR/2 weeks	Renal function, CBC, Hgb/4 weeks
Gastric protection		All cases	All cases

ACS = acute coronary syndrome; BMS = bare-metal stents; CBC = complete blood count; GPI = glycoprotein IIb/IIIa inhibitors; Hgb = haemoglobin; IHD = ischaemic heart disease; INR = International Normalized Ratio; NOAC = newer, non-vitamin K antagonist, direct oral anticoagulant; OAC = oral anticoagulation; TT = triple therapy; UFH = unfractionated heparin; VKA = vitamin K antagonist

[&] In non-emergency PCI.

[°] Close (one to three or four days) to PCI.

[*] UFH, 30–50 U/kg; enoxaparin, 0.3 mg/kg.

[§] UFH, 70–100 U/kg; enoxaparin, 0.5–0.75 mg/kg.

[#] Depending on the type (BMS vs DES) of stent and/or clinical setting (stable IHD vs ACS) of PCI.

[^] Dabigatran, 110 mg twice daily; rivaroxaban, 15 mg once daily; apixaban, 2.5 mg twice daily.

[**] In ACS.

[$] May be considered in ACS when bleeding risk is high.

In case of life-threatening or clinically relevant bleeding, general measures to preserve adequate circulation (plasma expanders, blood transfusions, inotropic support) and local control of haemorrhage (endoscopic treatment, surgical haemostasis), as well as reversal of anticoagulation when indicated, should be associated with the measures outlined above.

4.4 Summary of the management recommendations

An overview of the overall peri- and post-procedural management preferences/recommendations for OAC patients undergoing PCI is outlined in Table 4.12.

Key Reading

Dans AL, Connolly SJ, Wallentin L, Young S, Nakamya J, Brueckmann M, Ezekowitz M, Oldgren J, Eikelboom JW, Reilly PA, Yusuf S. Concomitant use of antiplatelet therapy with dabigatran or warfarin in the Randomized Evaluation of Long-Term Anticoagulation Therapy (RE-LY) Trial. *Circulation* 2013; **127:** 634–40.

Dewilde WJ, Oirbans T, Verheugt FW, Kelder JC, DeSmet BJ, Herrman JP, Adriaenssens T, Vrolix M, Heestermans AA, Vis MM, Tijsen JG, van't Hof AW, Ten Berg JW; for the WOEST study investigators. Use of clopidogrel with or without aspirin in patients taking oral anticoagulant therapy and undergoing percutaneous coronary intervention: an open-label, randomised, controlled trial. *Lancet* 2013; **381:** 1107–15.

Gao F, Zhou JY, Wang ZJ, Shen H, Liu XL, Nie B, Yan ZX, Yang SW, Jia DA, Yu M. Comparison of different antithrombotic regimens for patients with atrial fibrillation undergoing drug-eluting stent implantation. *Circ J* 2010; **74:** 701–8.

Lahtela H, Rubboli A, Schlitt A, Karjalainen PP, Niemelä M, Vikman S, Puurunen M, Weber M, Valencia J, Biancari F, Lip GY, Airaksinen KE for the AFCAS (Management of patients with Atrial Fibrillation undergoing Coronary Artery Stenting) study group. Heparin bridging vs. uninterrupted oral anticoagulation in patients with atrial fibrillation undergoing coronary artery stenting. *Circ J* 2012; **76:** 1363–8.

Lip GY, Huber K, Andreotti F, Arnesen H, Airaksinen KJ, Cuisset T, Kirchhof P, Marín F; European Society of Cardiology Working Group on Thrombosis. Document reviewers: Rubboli A, Camm AJ, Heidbuchel H, Hoffmann E, Reifart N, Ribichini F, Verheugt F. Management of antithrombotic therapy in atrial fibrillation patients presenting with acute coronary syndrome and/or undergoing percutaneous coronary intervention/stenting. *Thromb Haemost* 2010; **103:** 13–28.

Rubboli A, Halperin JL, Airaksinen KE, Buerke M, Eeckhout E, Freedman SB, Gershlick AH, Schlitt A, Tse HF, Verheugt FW, Lip GY. Antithrombotic therapy in patients treated with oral anticoagulation undergoing coronary artery stenting. An expert consensus document with focus on atrial fibrillation. *Ann Med* 2008; **40:** 428–36.

Rubboli A, Kovacic JC, Mehran R, Lip GY. Coronary stent implantation in patients committed to long-term oral anticoagulation therapy. Successfully navigating the treatment options. *Chest* 2011; **139:** 981–7.

Ruiz-Nodar JM, Marìn F, Roldàn V, Valencia J, Manzano-Fernàndez S, Caballero L, Hurtado JA, Sogorb F, Valdès M, Lip GY. Should we recommend oral anticoagulation therapy in patients with atrial fibrillation undergoing coronary artery stenting with a high HAS-BLED score? *Circ Cardiovasc Interv* 2012; **5:** 459–66.

Sarafoff N, Martischnig A, Wealer J, Mayer K, Mehilli J, Sibbing D, Kastrati A. Triple therapy with aspirin, prasugrel, and vitamin K antagonists in patients with drug-eluting stent implantation and an indication for oral anticoagulation. *J Am Coll Cardiol* 2013; **61:** 2060–6.

Schlitt A, Rubboli A, Lahtela H, Valencia J, Lip GY, Karjalainen PP, Weber M, Laine M, Kirchhof P, Niemelä M, Vikman S, Buerke M, Airaksinen KE for the AFCAS (Management of patients with Atrial Fibrillation undergoing Coronary Artery Stenting) study group. The management of patients with atrial fibrillation undergoing percutaneous coronary intervention with stent implantation: in-hospital data from the Management of patients with Atrial Fibrillation undergoing Coronary Artery Stenting (AFCAS) registry. *Catheter Cardiovasc Interv* 2013; **82:** E864–70.

Chapter 5

Essential pharmacology of antithrombotic agents

Thomas Cuisset, Stefan K. James, Andrea Rubboli, Lars
H. Rasmussen, Giancarlo Agnelli, Gregory Y. H. Lip

Key points

- Aspirin is a relatively weak antiplatelet agent, which acts through the irreversible inhibition of the platelet enzyme cyclo-oxygenase-1.
- $P2Y_{12}$-receptor inhibitors, including thienopyridines clopidogrel and prasugrel and cyclopentyl-triazolo-pyrimidine ticagrelor, are potent oral antiplatelet agents.
- Among parenteral anticoagulants, subcutaneous low-molecular-weight heparin, enoxaparin, and fondaparinux and intravenous bivalirudin have a superior efficacy-to-safety relationship.
- Vitamin K antagonists act by impairing the hepatic synthesis of coagulation factors II (prothrombin), VII, IX, and X and are complex to manage.
- Newer, non-vitamin K antagonist, direct oral anticoagulants inhibit single coagulation factors (thrombin, factor Xa) and have predictable anticoagulant effects with no need for routine laboratory monitoring.

Platelets and coagulation factors participate in the formation of thrombi at the arterial and venous sites. Whereas platelets activate and aggregate at the injured site following the exposure of extracellular matrix, small amounts of thrombin (factor IIa), which induce platelet activation and aggregation and promote activation of coagulation factors V, VII, and XI on platelet surfaces, are generated following the exposure to plasma of tissue factor-expressing cells. Intrinsic tenase and prothrombinase complexes are then formed, producing a burst of thrombin and the cleavage of fibrinogen to fibrin.

Because of the above mechanisms, administration of antiplatelet and/or anticoagulant drugs is required for effective antithrombotic treatment (Figure 5.1).

5.1 Antiplatelet drugs

5.1.1 Aspirin (Table 5.1)

By irreversibly inhibiting the platelet enzyme cyclo-oxygenase (COX)-1, aspirin blocks the conversion of arachidonic acid into prostaglandin-H_2 and therefore the formation

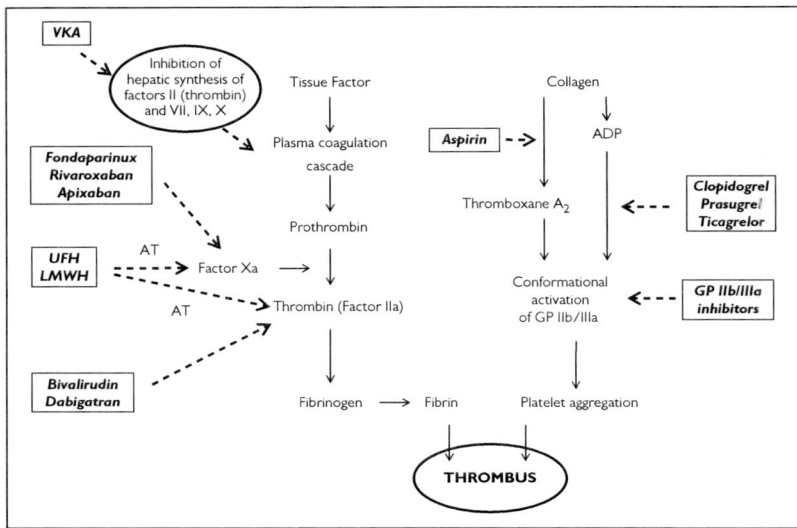

Figure 5.1 Pathways of thrombus formation, and action of antithrombotic drugs.
ADP = adenosine diphosphate; AT = antithrombin; GP = glycoprotein; LMWH = low-molecular-weight heparin; UFH = unfractionated heparin; VKA = vitamin K antagonist.

Table 5.1 Pharmacology of aspirin	
Prodrug	No
Target	Platelet COX-1 enzyme
Inhibition of target	Irreversible
Loading dose	150–325 mg PO (80–150 mg IV)
Maintenance dose	75–100 mg/day
Time to peak concentration	30–40 min (non-enteric-coated)
	3–4 h (enteric-coated)#
Plasma half-life	15–20 min
Bioavailabilty	40–50% PO (non-enteric-coated)
Onset of effect*	1 h
Duration of effect	3–4 days
Posology	OD
Relevant adverse effects	Dyspepsia
Discontinuation before surgery	Not required
Strategy for reversal	Discontinue; platelet transfusion

COX = cyclo-oxygenase; IPA = inhibition of platelet aggregation; IV = intravenous; OD = once daily; PO = orally
# Chewing is necessary when rapid effect is needed.
* Intended as time to IPA = 50%.

of thromboxane-A_2 (of which prostaglandin-H_2 is the immediate precursor), promoting platelet aggregation. Prostaglandin-H_2 is also the precursor of prostacyclin, which is produced by endothelial cells, and inhibits platelet aggregation. Aspirin is also able to inhibit COX-2 in endothelial cells, monocytes, and newly formed platelets, thereby blunting the anti-inflammatory response.

Nearly complete inhibition of platelet COX-1 can be achieved with aspirin doses of 75–100 mg/day. Because thromboxane-A_2 is largely derived from platelet COX-1, its formation is highly sensitive to aspirin, whereby prostacyclin formation is relatively insensitive to low-dose aspirin, as it is mainly dependent on COX-2 activity. Accordingly, residual COX-2–dependent prostacyclin biosynthesis is detected during low-dose aspirin treatment, whereas greater suppression of prostacyclin formation (and associated increased risk of thrombosis) may be observed with higher doses of aspirin (as well as with selective COX-2 inhibitors).

Aspirin is rapidly absorbed in the stomach and upper intestine. Plasma peak concentrations are reached rapidly after ingestion. Despite aspirin's short plasma half-life, the inhibition of platelet aggregation (IPA) persists for the platelet lifespan (about 10 days) because COX-1 inhibition is irreversible. After stopping aspirin, platelet function recovers faster (within three to four days) than predicted based on platelet turnover because the relationship between COX-1 inhibition and thromboxane-A_2 formation is non-linear.

Aspirin doses >50–100 mg/day do not increase IPA, whereas they may increase the risk of (gastrointestinal) bleeding. Such risk appears dose-dependent and is partly related to the direct toxic effect of aspirin (an acid) and partly to the reduced protective effect mediated by prostaglandins (inhibition of gastric acid secretion, regulation of gastric mucosal blood flow, mucus production).

Approximately 5% of patients treated with aspirin demonstrate high on-treatment platelet reactivity (HTPR; also defined as nonresponsiveness) and are at increased risk of thrombotic events. Whereas the pathophysiological mechanisms of HTPR are incompletely defined, there is no evidence that increasing the dose is of any benefit in patients experiencing a thrombotic event while on aspirin.

5.1.2 P2Y$_{12}$-receptor inhibitors (Table 5.2)

By binding to the P2Y$_{12}$-receptor on the platelet surface, these drugs inhibit adenosine diphosphate (ADP)-dependent platelet activation and aggregation, with no direct effects on the arachidonic acid pathway. They include the thienopyridines ticlopidine, clopidogrel, and prasugrel, and the cyclopentyl-triazolo-pyrimidine ticagrelor.

The first-generation thienopyridine *ticlopidine* has almost entirely been replaced by the second-generation clopidogrel because of a superior safety profile (no bone marrow toxicity).

Clopidogrel is an inactive prodrug, which undergoes rapid absorption after ingestion. Eighty-five per cent of the prodrug is hydrolysed by blood esterases to an inactive carboxylic acid derivative, whereas the remaining 15% is metabolized by the hepatic cytochrome P450 (CYP) 2C19 and 3A4 isoenzymes to the thiol derivative active metabolite. The active metabolite rapidly and irreversibly binds to the platelet P2Y$_{12}$-receptor, thus determining IPA for the lifespan of the platelets (about 10 days).

Dose-dependent IPA is seen after single oral doses of clopidogrel, with maximal platelet inhibition attained within four to six hours with a 300 mg loading dose and two to three hours with a 600 mg loading dose.

HTPR has been reported for approximately one-third of patients on clopidogrel. Whereas tests and cut-offs used to define HTPR may impact on the prevalence of this

Table 5.2 Pharmacology of P2Y$_{12}$-receptor inhibitors

Drug	Clopidogrel	Prasugrel	Ticagrelor
Class	Thienopyridine	Thienopyridine	Cyclopentyl-triazolo-pyrimidine
Prodrug	Yes	Yes	No
Receptor binding	Irreversible	Irreversible	Reversible
Loading dose	300/600 mg	60 mg	180 mg
Maintenance dose	75 mg/day	10 mg/day*	90 mg x 2/day
Time to peak concentration	1 h	30 min	1.5–3 h
Plasma half-life	8 h	7 h	8 h
Bioavailability	15%	80%	36%
Onset of effect#	4–6 h&/2–3 h§	30 min	40 min
Duration of effect	5–7 days	5–9 days	3–4 days
Maximum IPA	50–70%	80%	90%
Posology	OD	OD	BID
Relevant adverse effects:	—	—	Dyspnoea, bradyarrhythmias
Discontinuation before surgery	5 days	7 days	5 days
Strategy for reversal	Discontinue; platelet transfusion	Discontinue; platelet transfusion	Discontinue

BID = twice daily; IPA = inhibition of platelet aggregation induced by adenosine diphosphate; OD = once daily
TIA = transient ischaemic attack

* In patients at increased bleeding risk, 5 mg/day is advised.

Intended as time to IPA = 50%.

& Loading dose = 300 mg.

§ Loading dose = 600 mg.

patient subset, insufficient generation of the active metabolite is also of importance. Because of the complex (two-step) metabolic activation of clopidogrel, substances that inhibit CYP, including CYP3A4-metabolized statins (atorvastatin) or calcium-channel blockers (verapamil, diltiazem), and CYP2C19-metabolized proton-pump inhibitors (PPI; omeprazole, esomeprazole), as well as genetic polymorphisms in CYP, may be associated with a reduced laboratory response to clopidogrel. Whether these pharmacodynamic interactions have clinical relevance remains uncertain. At present, routine laboratory testing of clopidogrel response is not recommended, nor it is recommended to tailor therapy (increase of clopidogrel dose, or switching to newer P2Y$_{12}$-receptor inhibitors prasugrel or ticagrelor) based on platelet-function testing.

Prasugrel is a third-generation thienopyridine, which irreversibly binds to the platelet P2Y$_{12}$-receptor. IPA is greater with prasugrel compared to clopidogrel. Similar to clopidogrel, prasugrel is a prodrug requiring metabolic activation to exert its effect. After ingestion and rapid absorption, prasugrel is rapidly hydrolysed in the intestine, liver, and plasma to a thiolactone, which is then converted to the active metabolite by a single CYP-dependent step, primarily by CYP3A4 and CYP2B6. Approximately two-thirds of the prasugrel dose is excreted in the urine and approximately one-third in the faeces as inactive metabolites.

No significant interaction on prasugrel pharmacokinetics is to be expected by age, gender, and mild-moderate renal or hepatic impairment. Neither the inhibitors CYP3A4 (ketoconazole, verapamil, diltiazem, indinavir, clarithromycin, grapefruit juice), nor the inducers of CYP3A4 and CYP2B6 (rifampicin) are expected to significantly affect the pharmacokinetics of prasugrel. Concomitant administration of PPI or other drugs elevating gastric pH, or CYP3A4-metabolized atorvastatin, is not expected to have a significant effect on prasugrel metabolism either. No influence of the CYP genotype on prasugrel pharmacokinetics and pharmacodynamics has been shown. As a result, prasugrel treatment induces more consistent and less variable IPA, with an extremely low prevalence of subjects displaying HTPR.

Ticagrelor is a $P2Y_{12}$-receptor inhibitor of the class cyclopentyl-triazolo-pyrimidine. Unlike other $P2Y_{12}$-receptor inhibitors, ticagrelor does not need metabolic activation to exert its effect, and its binding to the $P2Y_{12}$-receptor is reversible. After ingestion and rapid absorption, however, ticagrelor is metabolized in the liver by CYP isoenzymes, mainly CYP3A4, to an active metabolite, which has a plasma concentration up to one-third that of the parent compound. Ticagrelor-induced IPA is stronger, faster, and more consistent than that induced by clopidogrel. Following drug cessation, effective IPA vanishes in three to four days, and after 24 hours from the last ticagrelor dose, the IPA is comparable to that of clopidogrel.

Because of the involvement of CYP isoenzymes, mainly CYP3A4, in the hepatic metabolism of ticagrelor, strong inhibitors of CYP3A4, including azole antimycotics (ketoconazole, itraconazole), HIV protease inhibitors (ritonavir, atazanavir), and clarithromycin, should be avoided because of the associated increased exposure to the drug. Potent CYP3A4 inducers, including simvastatin, rifampicin, dexamethasone, phenytoin, and carbamazepine, should be avoided as well because of the associated risk of reduced drug exposure.

Of importance, the maintenance dose of aspirin should not exceed 100 mg/day when given together with ticagrelor, as reduced effectiveness of ticagrelor has been observed with higher aspirin doses.

5.1.3 Glycoprotein IIb/IIIa inhibitors (GPI; Table 5.3)

The drugs of this class bind to the platelet glycoprotein IIb/IIIa receptor, which is a member of the integrin family of adhesion receptors and the common final step in the pathway that leads to platelet aggregation. By preventing the binding of fibrinogen to glycoprotein IIb/IIIa receptors of activated platelets, GPI inhibit platelet aggregation, irrespective of the metabolic pathway (arachidonic acid, ADP) responsible for initiating platelet aggregation. Currently, three GPI, namely abciximab, eptifibatide, and tirofiban, are available for intravenous (IV) only administration.

Abciximab is the antigen binding fragment of the chimeric human-murine monoclonal antibody against the platelet glycoprotein IIb/IIIa receptors. Bolus doses of abciximab induce almost full IPA (<20% of baseline). The onset of the antiplatelet effect appears within 10 min of administration, but the effect is temporary because abciximab plasma concentrations decrease rapidly (as a consequence of the rapid binding to glycoprotein IIb/IIIa receptors). Constant free plasma concentrations of abciximab, and sustained antiplatelet effect, are obtained with continuous infusion following IV bolus administration. At the termination of infusion, platelet function generally recovers over 24–48

Table 5.3 Pharmacology of intravenous GPI

	Abciximab	Eptifibatide	Tirofiban
Type	Monoclonal antibody fragment	Small molecule (cyclic peptide)	Small molecule (non-peptide)
Reversibility of binding	No	Yes	Yes
Platelet affinity	High	Low	High
Plasma half-life	10–30 min	2.5 h	2 h
Recovery of platelet function	Slow (24–48 h)	Fast (4 h)	Fast (4–8 h)
Route of elimination	Platelet binding	Renal (60–70%),	Renal (95%)
	Proteolytic cleavage	Biliary (20–30%)	
Renal dose adjustments	None	Yes*	Yes§
Dosing	0.25 mg/kg bolus + 0.125 mcg/kg/min for 12 h	180 mcg/kg bolus# + 2.0 mcg/kg/min for 18–24 h	25 mcg/kg IV bolus + 0.15 mcg/kg/min for 18–24 h
Strategy for reversal	Discontinue; platelet transfusion	Discontinue	Discontinue

CrCl = creatinine clearance; GPI = glycoprotein IIb/IIIa inhibitors

In the setting of percutaneous coronary intervention, a second 180 mcg/kg bolus is given 10 min after administration of the first bolus.

* When CrCl = 30–50 ml/min: 180 mcg/kg bolus + 1.0 mcg/kg/min infusion.

§ When CrCl is ≤30 ml/min: bolus and maintenance dose to be decreased by 50%.

hours, although abciximab remains in the circulation for ≥15 days in a platelet-bound state. Abciximab has been shown to elicit an antibody response, particularly after re-administration, thereby increasing the risk of thrombocytopaenia.

Eptifibatide is a synthetic cyclic heptapeptide mimicking a snake venom disintegrin, with high specificity for glycoprotein IIb/IIIa receptors. Eptifibatide is a competitive inhibitor of glycoprotein IIb/IIIa receptors, and nearly complete IPA (<20% of baseline) is observed immediately after IV bolus administration. Owing to the short half-life, continuous IV infusion is required to maintain sustained antiplatelet effect. Platelet function returns to baseline (>50% of platelet aggregation) after 4 h from stopping IV infusion. As eptifibatide is largely excreted by the kidney, dose adjustment and abstention from use are required in the presence of moderate and severe renal impairment, respectively. Albeit reported, the occurrence of thrombocytopaenia with eptifibatide is rare.

Tirofiban is a non-peptide, competitive inhibitor of platelet glycoprotein IIb/IIIa receptors. After IV bolus administration, almost complete IPA (<10% of baseline) is achieved. Because of the short half-life, continuous IV infusion is required to maintain sustained antiplatelet activity. Following discontinuation of infusion, platelet function recovers within 4–8 hours. Approximately two-thirds of tirofiban is excreted in urine, and therefore dose adjustment is warranted when severe renal impairment is present. As with other GPI, thrombocytopaenia has also been reported in patients receiving tirofiban.

5.2 **Anticoagulant drugs**

Anticoagulants can be classified as: a) parenteral (IV or subcutaneous (SC)), including unfractionated heparin (UFH), low-molecular-weight heparins (LMWH), fondaparinux, and bivalirudin; and b) oral, including vitamin K antagonists (VKA; warfarin, acenocoumarol, phenprocoumon), and newer, non-VKA, direct oral anticoagulants (NOAC; dabigatran, rivaroxaban, apixaban). All anticoagulants act by inhibiting either thrombin (factor IIa) action or generation.

Table 5.4 Pharmacology and management of parenteral anticoagulants

	UFH	LMWH (Enoxaparin)	Fondaparinux
Molecular weight (Daltons)	15,000 mean (range 3,000–30,000)	4,500 mean (range 2,000–9,000)	1,728
Average saccharide units	45	15	5
Main effects	Inactivation of thrombin, and factor Xa	Inactivation of factor Xa	Inactivation of factor Xa
Anti-Xa: antithrombin activity	1:1	3:1	—
Route of administration	IV/SC	IV/SC	SC
Plasma half-life (h)	1*	4–7	17
Bioavailability (%)	30	90	100
Time to peak concentration (h)	2–4	3–5	2
Monitoring	aPTT/ACT	anti-factor Xa activity#	anti-factor Xa activity#
Therapeutic dose	70–100 U/kg bolus	1 mg/kg BID SC	2.5 mg ACS
	12–18 U/kg/min infusion	1.5 mg/kg OD	5, 7.5,10 mg VTE$
		30 mg IV bolus +1 mg/kg SC BID	
Renal dose adjustments	No	Yes§	Yes^
Antidote	Protamine sulphate&	Protamine sulphate&°	None
Relevant adverse effects:	HIT, osteoporosis	—	—

ACS = acute coronary syndromes; ACT = activated clotting time; aPTT = activated partial thromboplastin time; BID = twice daily; HIT = heparin-induced thrombocytopaenia; IV = intravenous; SC = subcutaneous; OD = once daily; VTE = venous thromboembolism

* At conventional doses of approximately 100 U/kg.

Not routinely required.

$ For body weight <50 kg, 50–100 kg, >100 kg, respectively.

§ When creatinine clearance (CrCl) <30 ml/min: 1 mg/kg once daily instead of twice daily, or 1 mg/kg once daily instead of 1.5 mg/kg once daily; when CrCl = 30–80 ml/min: no dose adjustment, but clinical monitoring advised.

^ When CrCl <20 ml/min: contraindicated; 20–50 ml/min: dose to be reduced to 1.5 mg OD.

& Dose 1 mg/100 U.

° Partially effective (≤60%).

Table 5.5 Pharmacology and management of bivalirudin	
Class	Direct thrombin inhibitor
Target	Thrombin
Administration	IV
Bioavailability	100%
Plasma half-life	25 min
Renal dose adjustment	Yes#
Dose	0.75 mg/kg bolus + 1.75 mg/kg/h infusion§
Antidote	None
Relevant adverse effects:	—

IV = intravenous

When creatinine clearance (CrCl) <30 ml/min: contraindicated; 30–60 ml/min: reduced infusion dose of 1.4 mg/kg/h.

§ For at least the duration of procedure and up to 4 h after procedure.

5.2.1 Parenteral anticoagulants (Tables 5.4, 5.5)

UFH is a heterogeneous mixture of sulphated polysaccharide chains, with different molecular weights, anticoagulant activities, and pharmacokinetics. The majority of its anticoagulant activity is mediated through binding to antithrombin (AT) and subsequent inactivation of a number of enzymes in the coagulation cascade, including factor IIa (thrombin) and factors Xa, IXa, XIa, and XIIa. Thrombin and factor Xa are the most sensitive to inactivation. Formation of the ternary complex UFH/AT/thrombin is necessary for inhibition of thrombin, whereas binding of UFH to AT only is sufficient to inhibit factor Xa bound to AT. Binding of UFH to AT occurs through a unique, high-affinity pentasaccharide sequence, which is present in only one-third of UFH molecules. It is only this fraction that is responsible for the anticoagulant activity of UFH. UFH chains consisting of ≥18 saccharide units, which correspond to a molecular weight of about 5,400 Daltons, are of sufficient length to bridge AT to thrombin. UFH chains of <18 saccharide units containing the unique pentasaccharide sequence can inhibit only factor Xa. Thrombin-induced platelet activation is inhibited by UFH, which however may induce platelet aggregation by binding to platelets.

Once UFH is in the circulation, a number of plasma proteins compete with AT for UFH bridging, thereby reducing its anticoagulant activity. This contributes to the variable anticoagulant response to UFH and to the phenomenon of UFH resistance. UFH also binds to endothelial cells, further complicating its pharmacokinetics. UFH is cleared through a combination of a rapid saturable mechanism (binding to endothelial cells) and a slower, first-order mechanism. When the cellular binding sites are saturated, UFH enters the circulation, where it is cleared more slowly through the kidneys. At therapeutic doses, UFH is largely cleared through the rapid, saturable mechanism. The complex kinetics of UFH renders the anticoagulant effect non-linear, with both the peak activity and the duration of effect increasing disproportionately with increasing doses.

Because the anticoagulant response to UFH varies among patients, UFH therapy is monitored by and the dose adjusted based on the results of the activated partial thromboplastin time (aPTT; target aPTT ratio 2.0–3.0 of control) or, when higher UFH doses are given to prolong aPTT to the point of becoming unmeasurable and unreliable (percutaneous coronary intervention (PCI), bypass surgery), by the activated clotting time (ACT; target 300–400 s).

LMWH are derived from UFH by chemical or enzymatic depolymerization and are about one-third the molecular weight of UFH. About one-fifth of LMWH chains possess the pentasaccharide sequence, and only this fraction has anticoagulant activity. Like UFH, LMWH produce the anticoagulant effect by activating AT and accelerating the rate at which it inhibits thrombin and factor Xa. Because only pentasaccharide-containing chains ≥18 saccharide units are of sufficient length to bridge AT to thrombin, about 50–75% of LMWH are too short to catalyse thrombin inhibition. In contrast, all pentasaccharide-containing LMWH chains have the capacity to inactivate factor Xa. Consequently, LMWH have a greater capacity to promote factor Xa than to promote thrombin inhibition and have an anti-factor Xa:antithrombin ratio of 2:1 to 4:1, depending on molecular weight distribution. In contrast, UFH has an anti-factor Xa:antithrombin ratio of 1:1. No significant effect on platelet aggregation is exerted by LMWH. LMWH are prepared using different methods of UFH depolymerization, and each has a unique molecular weight that endows it, at least to some extent, with distinct pharmacokinetic and pharmacodynamic (anticoagulant) properties. Consequently, commercially available LMWH, including enoxaparin, dalteparin, nadroparin, and tinzaparin, are not interchangeable on a one-to-one basis.

LMWH, of which enoxaparin is the most widely used, have pharmacokinetic advantages over UFH, including higher bioavailability after SC injection (better absorption of shorter chains), more predictable anticoagulant response (reduced affinity for binding to plasma proteins), longer half-life, and a dose-independent half-life (reduced binding to endothelial cells). LMWH are given in fixed or weight-adjusted doses, without monitoring. Monitoring, however, may be required in renal failure and pregnancy. LMWH are cleared by the kidneys, and therefore can accumulate with impaired renal function. When monitoring is required, the anti-Xa level should be measured (target anti-factor Xa activity for enoxaparin ≥0.7 U/ml 4 h after injection).

Fondaparinux is a synthetic analogue of the pentasaccharide sequence present in UFH and LMWH that mediates their binding to AT. Fondaparinux shares all the advantages of LMWH over UFH. However, in contrast to LMWH, fondaparinux only inhibits factor Xa. The specific anti-factor Xa activity of fondaparinux is about seven-fold higher than that of LMWH. After administration, fondaparinux is fully bioavailable. Fondaparinux is mostly (about 70%) excreted unchanged in the urine and should therefore not be given with severe renal impairment. Fondaparinux is given in fixed doses, without need for routine monitoring. When required, monitoring should be performed by measuring anti-factor Xa levels.

Bivalirudin is a synthetic direct thrombin inhibitor, interacting with both the active site and the substrate-binding site of thrombin. Once in complex with thrombin, bivalirudin is slowly cleaved, thereby restoring the active-site function (and the coagulant activity) of thrombin. Importantly, bivalirudin does not activate platelets. Bivalirudin does not bind to plasma proteins; therefore it produces a more predictable anticoagulant response than UFH and is removed by haemodialysis. Bivalirudin is partially (approximately 20%) excreted by the kidney, with the half-life being prolonged with renal impairment. Dose adjustments and careful monitoring are therefore required when renal function is reduced. No routine monitoring is needed. Switching from IV UFH or SC LMWH to bivalirudin should be performed at least 30 min and 8 h, respectively, after stopping these drugs.

5.2.2 Oral anticoagulants

VKA inhibit the synthesis of normally functioning vitamin K-dependent coagulation factors II (prothrombin), VII, IX, and X. By interfering with the liver enzyme vitamin

Table 5.6 Pharmacology and management of warfarin

Class	Vitamin K antagonist
Target	Coagulation factors II (prothrombin), VII, IX, and X
Bioavailability	>90%
Time to peak concentration	2–4 h
Half-life	36–48 h
Onset of effect	24 h
Peak effect	72–96 h
Dose	Average 5 mg/day (range 1–20 mg/day)
Steady state after dose change	7 days
Missed dose	To be taken as soon as possible on the same day
Relevant adverse effects:	—

K-epoxide reductase subunit C1 (VKORC1), which is key for the cyclic conversion of vitamin K to vitamin K epoxide, which in turn modulates the γ-carboxylation of gluta-mate residues on vitamin K-dependent proteins, VKA treatment results in the hepatic production of decarboxylated and partially carboxylated proteins with reduced coagu-lant activity. VKA also inhibit carboxylation of the natural anticoagulant proteins C and S, therefore having the potential to induce a procoagulant state upon VKA treatment initiation. Warfarin, acenocoumarol, and phenprocoumon are the VKA that are com-mercially available. Of them, warfarin is largely the most used (Table 5.6).

Warfarin is a racemic mixture of R- and S-enantiomers, which have different charac-teristics. The S-enantiomer exhibits two to five times more anticoagulant activity but is cleared more rapidly than the R-enantiomer (29 vs 45 h). After ingestion, warfarin is rapidly and completely absorbed in the gastrointestinal tract, with rapid attainment of peak plasma concentrations. In the blood, warfarin circulates bound to plasma pro-teins, mainly albumin. The anticoagulant activity of a single warfarin dose generally lasts two to five days and may become more pronounced as the effect of daily mainte-nance doses overlap, in accordance with the different half-lives of the affected vitamin K-dependent coagulation factors (4–6 h for factor VII, 24 h for factor IX, 48–72 h for factor X, and 60 h for prothrombin) and natural anticoagulant proteins (8 and 30 h for proteins C and S, respectively). Warfarin is almost entirely cleared by hepatic CYP metabolism, with CYP2C9 primarily metabolizing the S-enantiomer, and CYP1A2 and CYP3A4, the R-enantiomer. In the presence of variant CYP2C9 alleles (about 10% of Caucasians), clearance of the S-enantiomer is decreased, and the exposure may there-fore be increased. Also, polymorphisms in the gene for VKORC1 have been associated with variable warfarin dose requirements. Variants of the CYP2C9 and VKORC1 genes are primarily responsible for the variability in warfarin dose requirements. Numerous drugs and foods may interact with warfarin through pharmacodynamic (synergism, competitive antagonism) or pharmacokinetic (enzyme induction or inhibition) mecha-nisms. As a result, drug or food interaction may produce an increased risk of bleeding or, conversely, an increased risk of thrombosis/thromboembolism (Table 5.7).

Acenocoumarol and phenprocoumon share with warfarin mechanism of action, metabolism, and pharmacological interactions. Like warfarin, they exist as R- and

Table 5.7 Major drug and food interactions with warfarin

	Increase INR and/or bleeding risk	Decrease INR and/or increase thrombotic risk
Drugs	Allopurinol	Carbamazepine
	Amiodarone	Omeprazole
	Amlodipine	Phenobarbital
	Atorvastatin	Phenytoin
	Ciprofloxacin	Prednisone
	Diltiazem	Rifampicin
	Escitalopram	Sucralfate
	Fluconazole	St John's wort
	Ketoconazole	—
	Metronidazole	—
	Miconazole	—
	Norfloxacin	—
	Oral contraceptives	—
	Propafenone	—
	Ranitidine	—
	Ranolazine	—
	Sertraline	—
	Ticlopidine	—
	Verapamil	—
Food	Fish oil	Soy milk
	Mango	Avocado
	Grapefruit	Ginseng
	Ginkgo biloba	—
	Cranberry	—

S-enantiomers, with different characteristics. Acenocoumarol and phenprocoumon have shorter (8–11 h) and longer (6–8 days), respectively, half-lives compared to warfarin and may be considered when a shorter or longer, respectively, duration of the anticoagulant effect is advised.

Unlike VKA, NOAC directly block single, activated, coagulation factors thrombin (factor IIa) or factor Xa. NOAC are characterized by rapid onset and offset of action, low propensity for drug and food interactions, and predictable anticoagulant effects after fixed-dose administration, therefore requiring no routine laboratory monitoring. The NOAC currently approved for clinical use include the direct thrombin inhibitor dabigatran etexilate and the factor Xa inhibitors rivaroxaban and apixaban (Table 5.8).

Table 5.8 Pharmacology of currently approved NOAC

	Dabigatran etexilate	Rivaroxaban	Apixaban
Prodrug	Yes	No	No
Target	Factor IIa (thrombin)	Factor Xa	Factor Xa
Bioavailability (%)	6–7	80–100	60
Time to peak concentration (h)	1–2	2–4	3–4
Plasma half-life (h)	12–17	5–11	12
Unchanged drug renal excretion (%)	>80	33	27

NOAC = newer, non-vitamin K antagonist, direct oral anticoagulant

Dabigatran etexilate is a prodrug with no pharmacological activity (Table 5.8). After oral administration, it is rapidly absorbed and converted to the active metabolite dabigatran by esterase-catalysed hydrolysis in plasma and liver. Dabigatran is a potent, competitive, and reversible direct thrombin inhibitor. Both free thrombin and clot-bound thrombin are inhibited, as well as thrombin-induced platelet aggregation. Whereas dabigatran etexilate is not metabolized by hepatic CYP, and therefore no interaction is expected with related drugs, it is the substrate of the efflux transporter P-glycoprotein (P-gp). Strong P-gp inhibitors and inducers increase and decrease, respectively, dabigatran plasma concentrations, thereby increasing the risks of bleeding and thromboembolism (Table 5.9).

Attention, with or without dose adjustment, is advised in patients with moderate renal impairment (CrCl 30–50 ml/min) because of the prolongation of dabigatran plasma half-life (to approximately 18 h) and therefore the prolonged exposure to its anticoagulant effect. Renal function, expressed as CrCl (ml/min), and estimated by the Cockcroft-Gault formula

140 – age (years) × weight (kg) (× 0.85 if female)/72 × serum creatinine (mg/dl)

should be determined before starting treatment and at least once a year, or whenever a decline in renal function is suspected. Attention, with or without dose adjustment, is also advised in situations at increased risk of bleeding, including age ≥75 years, weight ≤60 kg, and concomitant use of antiplatelet or non-steroidal anti-inflammatory drugs.

The coagulation tests that can be used to measure the anticoagulant effect of dabigatran include: aPTT (qualitative assessment) and diluted thrombin time (Hemoclot; quantitative assessment).

Rivaroxaban is a highly selective, reversible, direct factor Xa inhibitor (Table 5.8). Inhibition of factor Xa interrupts the coagulation cascade downstream, therefore inhibiting the formation of thrombin. No direct antithrombin activity or antiplatelet action is exerted by rivaroxaban. Because absorption and bioavailability of rivaroxaban are increased in fed conditions, the drug should be taken with meals. Two-thirds of rivaroxaban is metabolized in the liver, and one-third is eliminated by the kidney as unchanged, active substance. Hepatic metabolization occurs through CYP-dependent and CYP–independent mechanisms, the former mainly involving the CYP3A4 isoenzyme. Concomitant use of strong CYP3A4 inhibitors, as well as of strong P-gp inhibitors, of which rivaroxaban is a substrate, should be carried out with caution (Table 5.9).

Table 5.9 Major pharmacological interactions of NOAC

	Mechanism	Dabigatran	Rivaroxaban	Apixaban
Not recommended	P-gp inhibitor; CYP3A4 inhibitor	Ketoconazole	Ketoconazole	Ketoconazole
		Itraconazole	Itraconazole	Itraconazole
		Dronedarone	Dronedarone	Dronedarone
		Clarithromycin	Clarithromycin	Clarithromycin
		Erythromycin	Erythromycin	Erythromycin
		Ciclosporin	—	—
		Tacrolimus	—	—
	P-gp inducer; CYP3A4 inhibitor	Ritonavir	Ritonavir	Ritonavir
	P-gp inducer; CYP3A4 inducer	Rifampicin	—	Rifampicin
		St. John's wort	—	St. John's wort
		Carbamazepine	—	Carbamazepine
		Phenytoin	—	Phenytoin
		Phenobarbital	—	Phenobarbital
Caution^	P-gp inhibitor	Verapamil*	Verapamil	Verapamil
		Amiodarone	Amiodarone	Amiodarone
		Quinidine	Quinidine	Quinidine
			Ciclosporin	Ciclosporin
		—	Tacrolimus	Tacrolimus
		—	Diltiazem	Diltiazem
	P-gp inducer; CYP3A4 inducer	—	Rifampicin	—
		—	St. John's wort	—
		—	Carbamazepine	—
		—	Phenytoin	—
		—	Phenobarbital	—
No relevant interactions	P-gp inhibitor, CYP3A4 inhibitor	Atorvastatin	Atorvastatin	Atorvastatin
	P-gp inhibitor	Diltiazem	—	—
		Digoxin	Digoxin	Digoxin
	GI absorption	PPI	PPI	PPI
		H$_2$–receptor blockers	H$_2$–receptor blockers	H$_2$–receptor blockers

CYP = cytochrome P450; NOAC = newer, non-vitamin K antagonist, direct oral anticoagulants; PPI = proton-pump inhibitors
^ Dose reduction to be considered; * dose reduction (110 mg twice daily) to be performed.

Table 5.10 Management of currently approved NOAC

	Dabigatran	Rivaroxaban	Apixaban
Dose	NVAF *: 110/150 mg BID	NVAF#: 20 mg OD; DVT/PE°: 15 mg BID x 3 weeks + 20 mg OD onwards	NVAF *: 5 mg BID
Dose adjustments	Age >80 yrs, concomitant verapamil: 110 mg BID Age 75–80 yrs, CrCl 30–50 ml/min, gastritis/GORD, high bleeding risk: 110/150 mg BID§	CrCl 15–49 ml/min: 15 mg OD	≥2 of age ≥80 yrs, weight ≤60 kg, creatinine ≥1.5 mg/dl: 2.5 mg BID
Missed dose	>6 h prior to next: take missed dose <6 h prior to next: omit missed dose	During 20 mg OD, >12 h prior to next: take missed dose <12 h prior to next: omit missed dose	>6 h prior to next: take missed dose <6 h prior to next: omit missed dose
		During 15 mg BID, >12 h prior to next: take both doses together <12 h prior to next: omit missed dose	
Interactions	Food: no	Food: no$	Food: no
	PPI: no	—	—
Relevant adverse effects	Dyspepsia	—	—
Renal contraindications	CrCl <30 ml/min	CrCl <15 ml/min	CrCl <15 ml/min
Antidote	None^	None^	None^

BID = twice daily; CrCl = creatinine clearance; DVT = deep vein thrombosis; GORD = gastro-oesophageal reflux disease; NOAC = newer, non-vitamin K antagonist, direct oral anticoagulant; NVAF = non-valvular atrial fibrillation; OD = once daily; PE = pulmonary embolism; PPI = proton-pump inhibitors; TIA = transient ischaemic attack; yrs = years

* Risk factor ≥1 : prior stroke/TIA, age ≥75 yrs, hypertension, congestive heart failure (NYHA class ≥2 or left ventricle ejection fraction <40%), diabetes.

Prior stroke/TIA or ≥2 risk factors: congestive heart failure (NYHA class ≥2 or left ventricle ejection fraction <40%), age ≥75 years, hypertension, diabetes.

° Treatment of DVT and prevention of recurrent DVT/PE following an acute DVT.

§ To be evaluated on an individual basis.

^ Prothrombin complex concentrates (PCC), activated PCC (FEIBA), and recombinant factor VIIa may be considered.

$ Absorption and bioavailability increased in fed conditions, and therefore drug to be taken with meal.

Both strong inhibitors of CYP3A4 and P-gp may increase the plasma concentration of rivaroxaban, thereby substantially increasing the risk of bleeding. An increased exposure to rivaroxaban, with an associated increased risk of bleeding, is also observed with renal function impairment.

The coagulation tests that can be used to measure the anticoagulant effect of rivaroxaban include the prothrombin time (PT; with neoplastin) and anti-factor Xa activity (for which, however, no standard for calibration is available).

Apixaban is a highly selective, reversible, direct factor Xa inhibitor, which inhibits free and clot-bound factor Xa, and thus the formation of thrombin (Table 5.8). No direct inhibition of thrombin is exerted, nor does it have a direct effect on platelet function. Absorption of apixaban is not influenced by food, and the drug may be taken with or without a meal. Whereas apixaban is eliminated through several routes, the main metabolic pathway is in the liver, mainly by CYP3A4 and CYP3A5. Apixaban also is a substrate for the efflux transport P-gp, so that apixaban plasma concentrations and associated risk of bleeding are influenced by strong inhibitors of CYP3A4, CYP3A5, and/or P-gp (Table 5.9). Reduced renal function is associated with a mild to moderate increase in apixaban plasma concentrations. Because no relevant effect on the relationship between plasma concentrations and anti-factor Xa activity has been shown for mild to moderate renal insufficiency (CrCl 30–80 ml/min), no dose adjustment is required.

No coagulation tests have been validated to measure the anticoagulant activity of apixaban, which however should be carried out by measuring the anti-factor Xa activity.

An overview of the management of currently approved NOAC is reported in Table 5.10.

Key Reading

Ageno W, Gallus AS, Wittkowsky A, *et al.* Oral anticoagulant therapy: Antithrombotic therapy and prevention of thrombosis, 9th ed: American College of Chest Physicians evidence-based clinical practice guidelines. *Chest* 2012; **141 (Suppl):** e44S–e88S.

Becattini C, Vedovati MC, Agnelli G. Old and new oral anticoagulants for venous thromboembolism and atrial fibrillation: a review of the literature. *Thromb Res* 2012; **129:** 392–400.

Eikelboom JW, Hirsh J, Spencer FA, Baglin TP, Weitz JI. Antiplatelet drugs: Antithrombotic therapy and prevention of thrombosis, 9th ed: American College of Chest Physicians evidence-based clinical practice guidelines. *Chest* 2012; **141 (Suppl):** e89S–e119S.

Garcia DA, Baglin TP, Weitz JI, Samama MM. Parenteral anticoagulants: Antithrombotic therapy and prevention of thrombosis, 9th ed: American College of Chest Physicians evidence-based clinical practice guidelines. *Chest* 2012; **141 (Suppl):** e24S–e43S.

Huisman MV, Lip GY, Diener HC, *et al.* Dabigatran etexilate for stroke prevention in patients with atrial fibrillation : resolving uncertainties in clinical practice. *Thromb Haemost* 2012; **107:** 838–47.

Pengo V, Crippa L, Falanga A, *et al.* Questions and answers on the use of dabigatran and perspectives on the use of other new oral anticoagulants in patients with atrial fibrillation. A consensus document of the Italian Federation of Thrombosis Centers (FCSA). *Thromb Haemost* 2011; **106:** 868–76.

Turpie AGG, Kreutz R, Llau J, Norrving B, Haas S. Management consensus guidance for the use of rivaroxaban – an oral, direct factor Xa inhibitor. *Thromb Haemost* 2012; **108:** 876–86.